NUTRIPUNCTURE

NUTRIPUNCTURE

Stimulating the Energy Pathways of the Body Without Needles

Patrick Veret, M.D.,
Cristina Cuomo,
Fabio Burigana, M.D.,
and Antonio Dell'Aglio, M.D.

Translated by Jon E. Graham

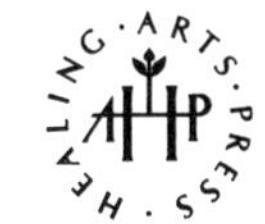

Healing Arts Press
Rochester, Vermont • Toronto, Canada

Healing Arts Press
One Park Street
Rochester, Vermont 05767
www.HealingArtsPress.com

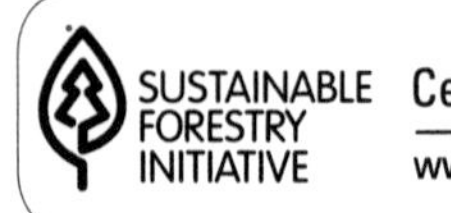

Text stock is SFI certified

Healing Arts Press is a division of Inner Traditions International

Originally published in French under the title *Méridiens et Nutripuncture: 39 nutriments essentiels à la vitalité de vos meridians* by Éditions du Dauphin, 43-45 rue de la Tombe-Issoire, 75014 Paris
First U.S. edition published in 2012 by Healing Arts Press

Note to the reader: This book is intended as an informational guide. The remedies, approaches, and techniques described herein are meant to supplement, and not to be a substitute for, professional medical care or treatment. They should not be used to treat a serious ailment without prior consultation with a qualified health care professional.

Library of Congress Cataloging-in-Publication Data is available

Veret, Patrick.
Nutripuncture : stimulating the energy pathways of the body without needles / Patrick Veret, Cristina Cuomo, Fabio Burigana, and Antonio Dell'Aglio.
p. cm.
Includes bibliographical references and index.
Summary: "A revolutionary nutrient therapy that stimulates the energetic pathways of the body to improve physical and psychological health—without needles"—Provided by publisher.
ISBN 978-1-59477-429-4 (pbk.)

Printed and bound in the United States by Lake Book Manufacturing
The text stock is SFI certified. The Sustainable Forestry Initiative® program promotes sustainable forest management.

10 9 8 7 6 5 4 3 2 1

Text design by Virginia Scott Bowman and layout by Priscilla Baker
This book was typeset in Garamond Premier Pro with Helvetica and Agenda used as display typefaces

To send correspondence to the authors of this book, mail a first-class letter to the authors c/o Inner Traditions • Bear & Company, One Park Street, Rochester, VT 05767, and we will forward the communication.

Contents

PART THREE

Targeted Action with Sequential Nutripuncture

FOREWORD

Patrick Veret's Breakthrough Science

By Edgar Morin

The originality of Patrick Veret's methods are a source of continued amazement to me and I am very inspired by the subject of this book, dedicated to assisting the body's own innate ability to maintain and increase its own vital potential.

Nutripuncture is a compilation of ideologies gathered from the biological, anthropological, and cosmic theories developed in traditional Chinese medicine, combined with informational and statistical concepts that have become more and more important in contemporary biology. In fact, research into life's fundamental organization, that of the cell, enables us now to describe in detail the notions of information and communication (between DNA via RNA proteins). DNA can be considered the patrimony of the human body's organizational memory with respect to the programs it automatically creates when stimulated by external activities.

The beauty of the art and science of Nutripuncture lies in the rich combination of a Western concept based on organic chemistry (molecules) with an Eastern concept, where the fundamental physical elements—Earth, Water, Air, Fire, Ether—are not broken down into their chemical compositions but rather seen as interacting freely with human beings in accordance with their more universal nature.

While Western philosophy tends to isolate individuals from their environment (natural, social, familial) and dissociate the body and mind, Eastern philosophy submerges them in a planetary world, at the heart of the cosmos, where they recognize the five elements and their active presence within the organism.

Furthermore, Nutripuncture incorporates the Chinese anatomical and physiological concepts of "meridians," invisible to conventional medicine's untrained eyes, but now, with the introduction of acupuncture, accepted in the West as viable pathways to release the unexplainable pain caused by both psychological and physical ailments.

Nutripuncture's uniqueness is the needle-free stimulation of the meridians; their healthy functioning is instead instigated by thirty-eight nutrients, taken in sequences of five. Over twenty-five years in existence, predominantly in European countries until recently, this marvelous science is merely in its infancy in its utilization as a viable and practical form of clinical practice. It has already proven to show positive results, although an infinite number of possibilities remain to be discovered.

Traditional Chinese doctors prevent diseases, as opposed to treating them, by frequently balancing bodily functions. In the same way, Nutripuncture's goals are to maintain an overall well-being so that disease and illness cannot invade our bodies. It is literally a "bodyguard," that protects our bodies against outside pathogens.

This bodyguard is simultaneously a parapet for the human mind, frequently under attack in today's fast-paced society by stressors and diverse challenges that are able to transform physical disorders into psychological ones and vice versa.

It is indisputable that Patrick Veret's research is a significantly important contribution to biological humanism.

EDGAR MORIN, a French sociologist and philosopher, is one of the most important thinkers of the current era. His interdisciplinary work attempts to understand the complexity of the world and the human being, to link knowledge, to overcome barriers and compartmentalization, while respecting the individual, biological, and cultural expression of the human, inseparable from the context in which it exists. Emeritus research director at the CNRS (French National Center for Scientific Research), president of the European Cultural Office (UNESCO), founder of the Association pour la pensée complexe (Association for Complex Thought), codirector of the Center for Interdisciplinary Studies (Sociology, Anthropology, Politics) at the Ecole des Hautes Etudes en Sciences Sociales (Grande Ecole for Social Sciences) (1973–1989), Edgar Morin is also a member of the Academic Council of the European Centre for Peace and Development at the United Nations University. His work has been translated into twenty-seven languages and is available in forty-two countries. His major work, *La Methode* (*Method*), is divided into six volumes.

PREFACE

Introducing the Authors

PATRICK VERET, M.D.

Life is full of unforeseen developments and chance encounters. If someone had told me when I was in medical school that I would do research on the body's vital currents, I would certainly have doubted them. In fact, at that time I was fascinated by surgery, as this branch of medicine has a rational aspect that always gave me reassurance. Furthermore, I had the good fortune to practice it during an internship in Neuilly under the guidance of a Parisian supervisor.

My internship was a very rewarding experience, which allowed me to realize that many clinical manifestations still escaped the explanations achieved by academic Cartesian reasoning, guided by the dogmas of linear thinking. In reality, confronted by a large number of disorders affecting a patient, the doctor often finds himself helpless: the tests are all normal yet the disorders are real, even though they cannot be placed in any clearly defined category.

During this time I had a cousin with many health issues and, as a young doctor, I was sure I could help him effectively. After many trials and errors, it was only homeopathy that permitted him to overcome his problems. My studies had given me no training in this discipline, which at first glance I found truly strange. I wondered, and I still wonder, how such weak dilutions can have any effect, especially when observing their results—which can be truly amazing—on animals.

In order to better grasp a practice that I found completely irrational, I began taking courses in homeopathy and spending time in a department where acupuncture was practiced. My meeting with a brilliant homeopathic physician let me grasp the tropism (movement in the direction of a stimulus) that a even a weak plant dilution could produce. When we talk about tropism we are also talking about a target. This began to interest me but then I faced the question of how to make this information evident on the human level.

My later meeting with Dr. Paul Nogier, researcher in auriculotherapy, which is based on the correspondence between the acupuncture points on the ear and the whole body,[1] allowed me to grasp the body's response to certain stimuli and to conduct my investigations in a new way. As I learned to detect clinical microsigns, I began approaching my patients differently, which brought an advantage to my consultations. In addition to the standard medical approach, I looked for imbalances of an "informational" nature, by identifying the disorders that could affect the body's ability to regulate itself. I tried to understand the body's reactions to stimuli, whether from homeopathic dilutions or acupuncture needles at specific sites. This gave me the guiding thread that has always governed my work and research.

During this time I became aware that before clinically and biologically identifiable disorders manifest in a person, there are imbalances of an informational nature, and that it is essential to restore their balance. I recognized that the sole person who really knew his problems was the patient himself, as they were manifesting inside his body. I therefore sought to trace the effect of different remedies on each person's terrain, governed by his or her body's tendencies toward imbalance. Without knowing I was doing so, I had begun working on the vital currents of the body, currents I had no idea existed.

My research only truly took off when I met Serge Lakhovsky, the son of the famous George, and Professor Etienne Guillé, who was the central figure of a group of students and researchers. During this time I had begun working at Orsay University (Paris) to compare my approach with that of researchers in cellular biology. Becoming familiar with the work of Georges Lakhovsky, who discovered the relationship between cellular oscillation and metals, and that of Barbara McClintock, who discovered that the genome can mutate in relationship to an external environmental influence, provided me an extremely fertile avenue of thought on the impact of the environment on cellular equilibrium.

The effect of Lakhovsky's oscillating circuits fascinated me, in particular their effect on plants. In fact, all that was needed for an injected tumor (*tuberculum tumefaciens*) to not prove inevitably fatal to a *Pelargonium* was to wrap a polymetallic coil around it. If it was possible to increase the vital potential of a plant, why wouldn't it be possible to do the same for a human being? But what is true for a plant is not conceivable for a human organism, formed by different vital systems in constant interaction and connected by specific currents called *meridians*.

It was therefore necessary to find the means to regulate the circulation of the vital currents of the body. Etienne Guillé taught me a great deal about the information carried by trace metals, which allowed me to learn that their impact in the body depends first and foremost on the support materials with which they are combined. I started getting together for Wednesday work meetings with Etienne Guillé and Serge Lakhovsky (who Etienne called "the President"), which were extremely enriching. Etienne explained his theories about metals and the experiments he had performed using radioactive copper 64. Every week we dined at the home of an "alchemist" of cuisine where our discussions in a nice atmosphere allowed each of us to profit from the experience and ideas of the others. This was a real cultural immersion, an exchange through which we formulated working hypotheses.

In fact nobody discovers anything all alone, as it is clearly the interaction between various people that at a given moment can make you shout "Eureka, I've got it!" Moreover, you never come up with nothing, as everything exists. But at a given moment you are capable, thanks to the stimuli of the milieu with which you are interacting, of having an intuition, a hypothesis, which you can verify afterward. Our first study was on the stimulation of the double layer of the cellular membrane. Even as I shuttled between Orsay and my office, we made many attempts to discover a nutritional formula that would restore the dynamic balance of the cellular membranes. Then one day the formula was there. A pharmacist manufactured it for us, allowing us to experiment and compare our results with the researchers at Orsay. This was how the first element from the Nutri range was born, which was called Nutri Yin–Nutri Yang.

Next we began stimulating the Liver meridian, guided by the natural tropism of certain plants—like Celandine (*Chelidonium majus*) on the right lobe of the liver and Saint Benedict thistle on the left lobe—and the impact of certain metal combinations. Step by step we gradually developed a range of thirty-eight nutritional supplements, called Nutris, which impact all of the meridians. They have now been used for many years to support the circulation of the different vital currents.

During this period we had no idea of the language of the meridians. Our goal was to simply potentialize a circuit in order to give it more vital energy. We learned this language later when it became obvious that we needed to identify the meridians in order to explain the consistency that guided the interaction of each meridian, and the cooperation of each circuit for the purpose of sustaining the body's self-regulation. This consistency permits them to function independently while being part of the same unit.

It was thus starting in 1992 that the idea occurred to me of using the Nutris to coordinate the synergic activities of the body's meridians instead of stimulating each meridian separately. By using five Nutris in a specific order we stumbled upon a precise language, the language of the body. For a language to be valid, everyone must be able to understand it and it must be replicable. As our work progressed I realized that it was revealing a universal language with the power to reveal a body's potential. It is this potential that Nutripuncture makes it possible for us to discover.

For many years now a large number of practitioners in Europe and North America have been able to see the benefits of applying this knowledge. However, this approach still remains a source of amazement—even for me. In fact, thanks to this kit of thirty-eight nutritional supplements, the "tool box" of Nutripuncture, we have gradually been able to grasp the complexity of the body and the interaction of the different vital currents guaranteeing its self-regulation.

Research on the voice and singing has recently opened new horizons for Nutripuncture studies. I have eagerly accepted the task of organizing numerous seminars targeting those who make a living using their voices, to gain a better understanding of the body's sonorous potential and the environmental factors necessary for its expression.

It gives me great pleasure to share this book based on the research I've conducted for the past thirty years. Indeed, the research making it possible to perfect the tools of Nutripuncture began in 1980 when I became interested in the impact of certain trace elements on cellular vitality. Research on the many possible applications of Nutripuncture continues to evolve, steadily improving our understanding of our individual responses to the challenges of our environment. It is just one more step closer to understanding what it means to be human, and the man and woman of the future.

CRISTINA CUOMO

I have known about Nutripuncture since it was first introduced in Italy in the 1990s by the "pioneers" who had begun using it and discovering its benefits. Around the same time, I had decided to quit smoking and a Roman acupuncturist had suggested I take trace element tablets to counteract the difficulties I was experiencing in freeing myself from my slavery to nicotine. Surprised, but trusting, I tried them and it has been nineteen years now since I even dreamed of smoking a cigarette. Highly motivated by the success of this experiment, I became increasingly interested in figuring out the mechanisms of this method, propelled by the curiosity that has always compelled me to get my finger on anything that can help me blossom. This was how I began studying Nutripuncture.

Beginning in childhood I had constantly suffered from liver problems, which my mother, an allopathic doctor, treated with the standard medical remedies. However, my liver remained quite fragile, always ready to react adversely to a simple taste of Nutella or the merest upset. Like many others, I did not know just how bad I felt because I did not really know what it was like to "feel good." But when I began using Nutripuncture to dynamize my liver meridians, I was filled with a new energy. My newfound sense of well-being liberated me from the inner feelings of frustration that had been with me since I was small. I realized that the relationship between the mind and the body was a real one. One thing leading to another, I continued giving my cells a real boost by feeding my delicate vital currents. What happiness!

For many years now I have been a member of a French Italian multidisciplinary Nutripuncture research team, which has enabled me to learn many things. First and foremost is the fact that the body has an amazing ability to regenerate when the stimulations required for its self-regulation are available. I realized that cells are extremely intelligent (much smarter than me!), that they are always on the prowl for information, propelled by their ability to organize, cooperate, share, and exchange.

While I was studying for my degree in psychology at the university I often wondered why the body had always been overlooked and separated from the mind. The teaching I received, which was primarily based on theory, forgot the permanent interaction of the mind and body. There is nothing so surprising about this, as the body inspires fear. Tackling its knowledge, the massive amount of information it has recorded over millions of years of evolution, may well pose a challenge that can never be met. However, its knowledge and highly sophisticated programming permit it to constantly adapt and regulate itself, forming a resource as valuable as the knowledge science has amassed over several centuries.

Animated by the desire to rediscover the threads connecting the mind-body unit, I performed research for several years on the impact of babies' first movements on cerebral maturation, which allowed me to put my finger on the power of the body and its memories. This was how I learned that our brain, immature at birth, builds its neurological networks, thanks to the first movements performed by all babies in learning how to walk, and how its skills are aroused by sensorial information it receives from the environment.

Nutripuncture allowed me to realize that body memories are a precious legacy that can be learned with humility, without necessarily "understanding" them and dominating them, but simply acknowledging them. When the language life uses to express itself addresses you, your only response can be amazement!

After years of research and studies in nutrition, sports physiology, and psychology, I have become convinced that Nutripuncture is an excellent, simple, and effective method for activating the body's potential and enriching ourselves with the knowledge the body has etched in its memory banks. With ever-deepening respect, I continue to discover more about the amazing complexity of the human body, its memories, and its language, every day finding valuable benchmarks I consider as real wealth.

Although our process of writing this book has been a true birth labor, in which I had to face many questions and assume great responsibility, I am happy that today we can share it with all those seeking to advance toward self-awareness. This book makes available to both lay readers and practitioners high-performance tools for taking charge of their bodies and discovering their true potential.

All human beings, men and women alike, hold a great responsibility to themselves and all other forms of life: the choices we face are of fundamental importance for our own future and that of our planet. This is something that concerns each and every one of us: as we each take responsibility for our own well-being and psychophysical equilibrium, we take part in the overall health of the human community and our wonderful world.

FABIO BURIGANA, M.D.

A little more than ten years ago, a friend invited me to attend a seminar given by a French doctor who claimed he could stimulate the acupuncture meridians with trace element complexes. I had long contemplated deepening my knowledge of Eastern medicine, without seeking to become an acupuncturist, however.

My experience as a hospital practitioner in the field of gastroenterology, nuclear medicine, and internal medicine had already revealed to me both the benefits and limitations of contemporary medicine. The fact is, despite the undeniable advances in modern medicine, there still remains a large empty space that all "honest" doctors can see, a vacuum with consequences, the cost of which are paid by their patients. This large vacuum is probably the fruit of a lack of recognition of the life and unique personality of each and every individual who comes to us seeking aid.

I have personally always viewed medicine as a means of restoring the harmony necessary for us to live at our highest level and to express our personality. The fact that a doctor today is regarded as a "repairman for breakdowns" had already inspired me to look for answers in other medical perspectives such as homeopathy, osteopathy, and anthroposophical medicine.

After hearing Dr. Veret's presentation at his seminar, I realized that I had already integrated a number of things whose existence I had barely discovered. I was looking in the same direction but he was already seeing things much further ahead. His technique of Nutripuncture integrated Eastern tradition and homeopathy as well as the latest research in the fields of biology and physics, combined with ideas I had previously found only in the work of Rudolf Steiner. In addition to all this, he possessed the ability to observe, something I believe to be his most valuable and amazing quality.

For him, the voice, the glance, the posture, and everything else about a patient expresses the balance or imbalance of the vital currents that link his or her organs and connect him or her with the environment and the cosmos. This let me discover that Dr. Veret was a veritable artist, a master of the "art of medicine," capable of grasping these manifestations of life and, thanks to his technique, paving the way for extraordinary changes.

This first meeting prompted my decision to follow his teaching and combine Nutripuncture with the techniques I was already using in my work. In no time this new approach became a core and fundamental aspect of my professional activity, one that allowed me to obtain excellent results, even in some very complex situations.

At the same time, thanks to Dr. Veret's advice, I was beginning to use Nutripuncture to address my own health problems. Restoring new equilibrium to my vital currents not only solved my health issues but also increased my observational abilities and opened new horizons in my professional activity.

This is what led me several years ago to begin offering workshops intended for other health professionals as well as singers and actors and other people whose voice is their profession. At first perplexed by their introduction to the holistic approach of Nutripuncture, my students were soon amazed at the changes that could be seen and measured with different techniques in posture or simply by listening to the changes in vocal expression.

I noted that the students who grasped the full range of this discipline the fastest were osteopaths. By virtue of the sensitivity that is the distinctive feature of their practice, they were able to perceive the micro modulations that were occurring both on the level of the osteomuscular structure and the visceral level. They were sometimes astounded by the transformation they could see after stimulating their patients with Nutripuncture, whereas the majority of time, they had to perform several sessions before achieving the same results.

Normally the osteopath starts treatment by drawing up a complete diagnosis of the patient, then uses his or her hands to transmit the information needed to correct the dysfunction—just like Nutripuncture works using trace element complexes. In reality, these two disciplines, osteopathy and Nutripuncture, have a synergic effect and have proven to be quite complementary.

Training in Nutripuncture has until now been based on the notes and diagrams presented during courses, and the absence of a core reference work has been keenly felt. This is the reason why Cristina Cuomo, Antonio Dell'Aglio, and I decided to assemble Dr. Veret's central teachings in this one volume. Dr. Veret's collaboration has enabled us to better portray the basic tenets of Nutripuncture we are presenting here. It is my hope that this book will become a reference work for all those wishing to learn this incredible information approach to what it is to be human.

ANTONIO DELL'AGLIO, M.D.

During my professional life as a doctor of stomatology and orthodontics, I have been confronted by complex disorders affecting the mouth, whose solutions were often long and difficult. I was often perplexed by the various therapies learned in medical school and developed further with renowned international experts during my ongoing training. The gaps in the practical application of the theories and especially the lack of any research concerning the causes of pathological disorders affecting the mouth (teeth, gums, temporomandibular joint) always left me unsatisfied.

All I knew on this subject seemed insufficient and I felt a need to reconnect the mouth to the rest of the body, to restore it to its rightful place and reestablish its connections with the mind of the man or woman who visited my office for consultation.

This was what led me to seek out new approaches in the field of alternative medicine, albeit while still referring to all my scientific and medical school baggage. During this unrelenting quest, one I maintained unfailingly for many years, I came into contact with herbal therapy, flower therapy, and posturology, therefore increasing my baggage of knowledge. My discovery of Nutripuncture allowed me to look at my practice in a new light, to integrate a holistic vision of the human being, and, most importantly, to reconcile the scientific aspect with the humanist aspect of medicine.

My research into Nutripuncture helped me find countless answers to the questions I had long been asking myself about the origin of disease. To provide just a couple of examples:

Orthodontic treatments can easily regress if the vital currents involved are not supported by Nutripuncture.

All prosthetics, even if crafted perfectly, will be hard put to endure the severe treatment they are subjected to on a nightly basis by individuals afflicted with bruxism (the grinding of teeth). Rapid improvement will be seen when the vital currents involved are dynamized.

My "mechanical" activity as a doctor and orthodontist gradually evolved and—thanks to the systematic application of Nutripuncture—I learned how to restore balance to the cellular terrain and correct conditions that had been making the appearance of numerous mouth disorders possible.

Thanks to the application of this method, I discovered how the body can recover its sometimes amazing ability to regulate itself. By using and teaching Nutripuncture I also learned to see the human being in his or her integrity, incorporated within an immense and complex energy field, and subject (from the time of being an embryo) to the influence of the natural world and human relationships.

During many years of personal experience I have seen that Nutripuncture allows people to refine the perception of their own bodies, to better understand the impact of a dysfunction upon their overall psychophysical vitality, to expand their self-awareness and to learn just how we communicate with one another. Over this time I rediscovered the simple laws that govern the human being's equilibrium and I grasped the very intimate relationship that exists between behavior and physical disorders. This changed the way I performed my profession and the way I approached the people who came to me for consultation.

I am deeply and sincerely grateful to Dr. Veret, the primary researcher and father of Nutripuncture, for spreading this incredibly rich teaching that offers future researchers countless leads for future studies of human vitality. I was therefore extremely delighted to have this opportunity to take part in the writing of this manual.

Putting Nutripuncture into Practice

Please note, the authors cannot be held responsible for the consequences of any practice or misuse of the information contained in this book. The content of this book reflects the experiences and observations of the authors and should not be considered therapeutic advice. Any health problems should be treated by an appropriate professional health care practitioner.

Acknowledgments

A big thank-you to all the European and North American practitioners who have taken part in the many long years of Nutripuncture research and have thereby played a vital role in the perfection of its practical applications. Their collaboration made it possible to carry this study of human complexity much farther and to verify both its benefits and limitations.

Our special thanks to Andrew Heimann for his precious care in helping us to transmit and maintain the Nutripuncture spirit from French into English.

INTRODUCTION

What Is Nutripuncture?

A NEW APPROACH enabling the management of our vital potential in a simple and primal way, Nutripuncture stands at the crossroads of Western scientific knowledge, referenced in most recent biomedical discoveries, and thousands of years of knowledge from traditional Chinese medicine philosophy, which underlines the interaction between organism and environment.

Nutripuncture activates self-regulation, the body's own innate ability to optimally interact with its ever-changing environment (changes of season, stresses in life, relationship conflicts, and so on). When well-balanced vital currents nourish the body, we are better able to manage our emotions and achieve our sensory, creative, and cognitive potential.

Unfortunately, no matter how deeply we wish and no matter how enthusiastically we try, it is not always possible to use our body's potential to our best advantage. Despite the fact that we have at our disposal an organism that is among the most sophisticated nature has crafted over millions of years of evolution, we do not always know how to "drive" it appropriately, having misplaced the instructions. Today we know that we use only a minuscule part of our potential, probably because we are unaware of the elements governing the amazing complexity of organic life.

Life is an experience that each of us works out in accordance with our sensory vitality—the acuteness of our gustatory, auditory, olfactory, visual, and tactile receptors—which allows us to perceive all the nuances of reality. This is the basis for the relationship we maintain with our body.

From the time of birth, experience is fundamental to individual development and is an essential "fertilizer" for awakening the abilities programmed in the genes of every human being. In fact, without adequate stimuli, all the information contained in our gene pool cannot be activated. Light, for example, is essential to awaken the eye's visual potential, sounds are vital stimuli for developing the ears' capabilities, and so forth.

The various pieces of sensory information we receive from our environment, both natural and social, in their turn make it possible to organize a system of greater complexity, one that has not been programmed in our genes but is the fruit of our experience. This is our cognitive potential, another way of describing our personal capacity for integrating experience in accordance with the information we have received and selected.

This is how each human being builds him or herself in accordance with the quality and quantity of the stimuli received. If we can manage to acknowledge and integrate the information provided by our five senses, our experience will be positive and will nurture our growth. On the other hand, if we cannot manage to assimilate our experience or "turn it to our advantage," it will be perceived as stress and felt as a hindrance to our psychophysical evolution.

Personal development and individual initiative are the two faces of the new rule of today's social game, one that inspires an all-pervasive competition that can often be quite difficult to handle without adverse consequences. Our society, with its excessive emphasis on efficiency and its worship of achievement, conditions us to live with stress on a daily basis and accept it as normal. However, it has an enormous impact not only on our relationships with others but on our mental and physical vitality as well. It causes a reduction of our sensory perception and our brain's performance. Stress is our cells' worst enemy and is the source of a wide number of disorders that manifest in various ways, depending on the sensibility and biological terrain of the individual.

Some stress can be tied to childhood, but also to the death of a loved one, a physical or moral assault, the loss of a job, moving, an abortion, a divorce, and so on. All these trials leave their mark on the individual, becoming etched in memory and interfering with the harmonious circulation of the information the body requires for its self-regulation.

We can fight the consequences of stress with allopathic products like anti-anxiety drugs or antidepressants. Other therapies are also available, but they share the same goal of combating the symptom. For example, herbal medicine offers us

Stress Can Be Defined Both Quantitatively and Qualitatively

Quantitatively, stress involves a stimuli overload (a overly large quantity of information that the person cannot manage to integrate), or a lack of stimuli, which causes performance to regress.

Qualitatively, stress involves stimulations that have been voided of their content and contain no structuring information. For example, you may be eating enough but if the foods ingested are poor in nutrients, lack vitamins, or contain unhealthy fats, your cells will suffer from considerable oxidative stress. Or relationships that provide no real emotional exchange on the psychic level can also sometimes impose an unmanageable stress on the mind.

plants that target their effects on specific areas of the body. We can also turn to homeopathy or acupuncture, which can regulate energy flows in the body to deal with a specific symptom. Other natural approaches include shiatsu or Chinese massage, which work to bridge over the disorder that has manifested physically. There are other techniques such as sophrology, whose objective is to increase self-awareness, or hypnosis, for the treatment of pain and chronic stress. These are all ways of "fighting against" the symptoms of stress.

Psychologists take a primarily psycho-emotional approach to treating the individual, relying on the various theories emerging from this new science that was born little longer than a century ago. The different psychosomatic approaches call for study of behavior and the psyche without establishing precise cause and effect connections, and without necessarily connecting the mind to the body, which is the support of all human expression. However, an obvious connection exists between physical and mental disorders!

When illness appears, we can consider it as a failure of the body's natural ability to regulate itself, a loss of its natural or acquired immunity. It goes without saying that aid must be given the body by all the modern methods—allopathy, surgery, chemotherapy, and so on—in order to counter the development of a pathological condition. In tandem with this action, which fights against a symptom, we can also try to comprehend the deep causes for the disorder. They are often visible in the apparent relationships of cause and effect. When it is an infection, for example, generally a germ is the culprit. If it is malaria, we know the cause: mosquitoes and, of course, the humid environment that is favorable to their development.

In other areas, especially chronic disorders, there is no obvious answer on the causal level. We can sometimes mention several factors, once more demonstrating the complexity of human reactions to the environment. We can blame the gradual modification of the biological terrain, according to the milieu whose information has eventually become etched into the cellular level.

Today, numerous studies have finally demonstrated the interactions between the endocrine, nervous, and immune systems, and have proven the existence of a psycho-neuro-endo-immunological network (PNEI). Complexity research, tying together all the different kinds of knowledge viewed separately until now, also provides an overall look at the different facets of human expression, giving us a better grasp of the interactions between different physiological systems as well as the interactions between the organism and the environment. The individual is hence considered as an open system that is constantly interacting with its surroundings (natural, relational, and social).

Nutripuncture is consistent with these findings, as it is based upon a holistic vision of the human being, taking into account the various factors (internal and external) that can interfere with an individual's psychophysical vitality. The mindset animating Nutripuncture is completely different from all the others mentioned, as it never fights against a symptom but seeks to strengthen the body's natural ability to regulate itself so that it can recover its vitality. *Nutripuncture does not fight "against" stress, but is a means for stimulating our vitality.*

Inspired by the work of several scientists who were pioneers in their fields, and referring to the millennia-old laws of Eastern tradition, Nutripuncture was born as the result of research performed by numerous practitioners on the role played in the human dynamic by the vital currents. The vital currents, which flow along the lines known in acupuncture as *meridians,* stimulate the communication, cooperation, and coordination of all sectors of the organism (body), as well as the consistent operation required for the individual to adapt to the environment. Each meridian line in Nutripuncture is labeled by a number, from 01 to 38 (there are twenty-eight meridian lines for everyone plus five that are specifically male and five specifically female). When the circulation along the meridians is encouraged, the body is provided new impulses that reduce the impact of stress on our vitality and neutralize the information that has weakened our vital currents.

For this purpose Nutripuncture uses thirty-eight mineral complexes (Nutri 01, Nutri 02, Nutri 03, and so on), which stimulate the harmonious circulation of the vital currents via the meridian lines. Each mineral supplement, or Nutri, targets a specific meridian and bears the same number, from 01 to 38, as the meridian it targets. In addition to this range of thirty-eight specific Nutris, a General Cellular Nutritional Regulator (Nutri Yin–Nutri Yang) was created, which nourishes the cell membrane's activity, necessary for cellular exchanges, a true reflection of the organism's vitality.

It has long been known that minerals and trace elements are essential to cellular life. The Nutris are the concrete result of research performed on the action of trace minerals, often combined in accordance with complex protocols, on the circulation of the vital currents. In the 1980s, thanks to experiments at the University of Orsay in Paris, researchers discovered that when the minerals are combined in a specific sequence, the patterns created by these Nutris give life to a language, an alphabet, that the organism (body) recognizes and responds to in a coherent way. The synergy of the combined Nutris exhibits emergent properties that are not present in each component singly.

The effect of these trace elements is incisive and almost immediate. The ingested trace elements trigger, via the taste buds, an electromagnetic activity that encourages the circulation of the information necessary for our overall dynamic. In fact, the electromagnetic path, as opposed to the slower chemical path, uses very efficient transmitters that are incredibly fast: biophotons. These light particles, which play a role in the communication between cells, have been studied by expert researchers (F. A. Popp, V. L. Voeikov, and A. Gurwitsch[1]) who sought to gain a better understanding of light's role in the body, where it is involved in the regulation of biological functions and the coordination of cellular activities. By using the nutritional supplements, the Nutris, we have gradually acquired enough experience to refine

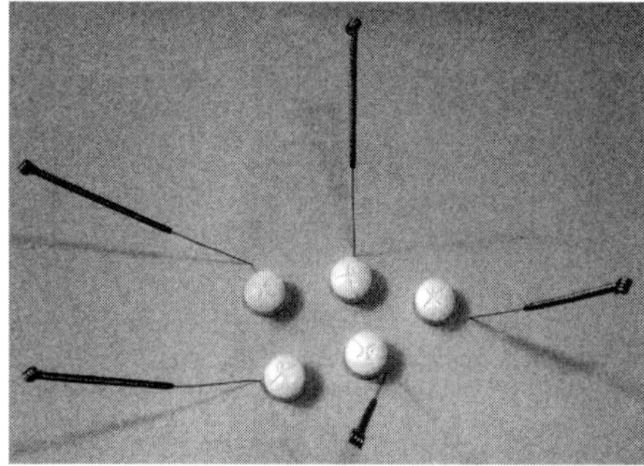

Fig. I.1. With Nutripuncture, trace element tablets are used instead of acupuncture needles

regulation of the vital currents and sharpen our knowledge of their role in individual psychophysical balance.

Nutripuncture offers the body the information it needs to carry out its dynamic processes and sharpen its sensory perception. In this way it encourages self-awareness, making it possible to discover our essential internal landmarks, which are indispensable references for communicating and interacting consistently with our social and natural environment. The expression used by Edgar Morin in his foreword, "bodyguard," is an excellent definition for the role and valuable services provided by this approach, an approach that is within the grasp of everyone.

In order to make the Nutripuncture approach fully accessible to all, our findings are presented in this book in three parts. Part 1 will provide you with the background and basics, which will make it clear that the research conducted on Nutripuncture offers a complete look at ourselves as human beings with physical and mental dimensions, providing us with a better grasp of the impact of stress on our overall equilibrium and the vital currents of the body. Thanks to the experience gained over the last ten years, particularly in the field of stress, we can evaluate the importance of the biological terrain and the major role of the meridians responsible for the circulation of the information necessary for the smooth unfolding of the passages marking the different stages of human development. We will explore the theory and practice of Nutripuncture, demonstrating how and why it is able to activate the vital potential of the organism (body), enabling it to reach maximum optimal vitality, and to ensure well-being. The different protocols that have been perfected for restoring greater vitality are described. A readily accessible application of Nutripuncture, attuning the dynamics of the vital currents to the rhythm of the seasons, is presented as an inviting introductory use of this knowledge.

Part 2 presents Associative Nutripuncture, a way of regulating the meridian lines, particularly in response to an occasional stress, momentary disturbance, or seasonal change, which makes it possible to regain better balance quickly. Initially the General Cellular Nutritional Regulator (Nutri Yin–Nutri Yang) is used, in combination with several Nutris chosen according to the meridian lines requiring regulation, because they show excess or deficient energy. This first approach is simple and within anyone's reach; it reinforces overall well-being and nourishes the terrain in which certain disorders can surface if left unchecked.

Part 3 presents Sequential Nutripuncture, which involves the simultaneous regulation of five meridian lines (without using the General Cellular Nutritional Regulator), combined according to a precise order (*sequence*), conveying specific information according to the mapped circuit in question. Indeed, each *sequence* is like a sentence made up of five words, which, according to their place, express different information. The sequence makes it possible to regulate each meridian line and each organ, and to enhance each function and dynamic, by respecting its uniqueness and incorporating it in the organism as a whole.

Research in Nutripuncture has produced an impressive portfolio of sequences, which have been adapted to the "language of the body" and confirmed by experiments. For example, it has been observed that one kind of stress (grief, for instance) weakens specific vital currents, which are always the same, although the way individuals react to a given event is completely personal. The activation of the thirty-eight meridians, stimulating five precise points each time, offers an incredible number of combinations defined in precise terms, making it possible to dynamize the vital currents that have been weakened by mental or physical stress.

The book is enhanced by three appendices. The first, appendix A, describes the benefits of using Nutripuncture to support human communication through movement, gesture, and the voice. Appendix B offers the reader who wishes to explore further a list of resources: sources for Nutris, practitioners, and teachers. Finally, the testimonials in appendix C make it clear that Nutripuncture is a powerful way to enhance the body's ability to regulate itself.

Today the World Health Organization (WHO) is increasingly interested in the vital equilibrium and dynamic of health. In its 1978 Alma Ata statement,

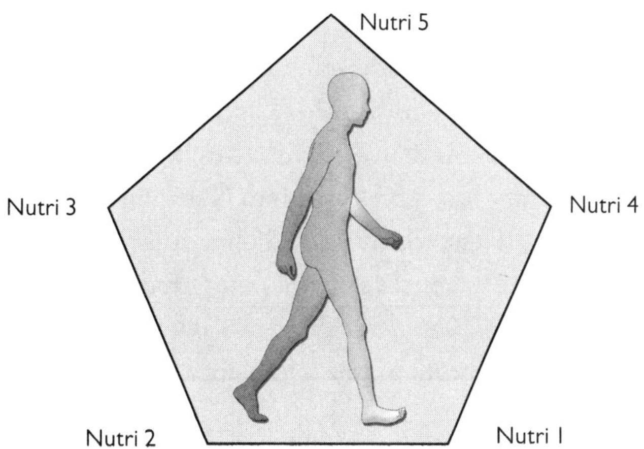

Fig. I.2. Sequential Nutripuncture is a language using phrases that always consist of five words, which target a specific circuit of meridians.

the WHO emphasized the importance of introducing complementary fields of medicine, whose effectiveness had been demonstrated scientifically, into the different national health care systems.

This approach was the subject of an international seminar held in October 2008 in Florence, Italy, on the theme "Innovation and Integration of Complementary and Traditional Medicines in Public Healthcare Systems." This meeting was organized by Tuscany, the first Italian region to integrate complementary techniques in its public health care system, which it had done several years earlier. We gave a presentation of Nutripuncture and its research during this seminar. The opening speech provided by Edgar Morin offered an ethical definition of research striving to capture human complexity through connecting the various domains of knowledge, and the importance of these studies.

The disparity of health problems around the world presented during this international gathering was particularly interesting. For example, in Bolivia, the objective of some NGOs was to reduce female mortality after birth from puerperal infections. The mortality rate was five percent; today it is two percent thanks to the courageous efforts of men and women working on behalf of a populace that is still mostly illiterate.

Conversely, in the Italian region of Tuscany, with its three million inhabitants, the yearly rate of medical visits is sixty million! Fortunately, the majority of these consultations do not involve life-threatening issues but are rather motivated by a sense of psychophysical discomfort that needs to be addressed to avoid the manifestation of more serious disorders.

It is in this particular domain of malaise, a general feeling of being unwell, that Nutripuncture has a significant role to play. On the one hand it represents a new approach to understanding the circumstances that are favorable for a symptom to appear. On the other hand, it offers "tools" to help us overcome the often difficult ordeals that we have to deal with at every age.

Twenty years of research into Nutripuncture has clearly shown that use of these thirty-nine supplements has allowed a large number of men and women to rediscover their essential reference points and gain a new lease on life. This book will allow you to discover the principles and many applications of this valuable approach. Then it will be up to you to decide whether you wish to try it for yourself.

PART ONE

Fundamentals of Nutripuncture

Man knows and his capacity to know depends on his biological integrity; furthermore, he knows that he knows. As a basic psychological and, hence, biological function cognition guides his handling of the universe and knowledge gives certainty to his acts; objective knowledge seems possible and through objective knowledge the universe appears systematic and predictable. Yet knowledge as an experience is something personal and private that cannot be transferred, and that which one believes to be transferable, objective knowledge, must always be created by the listener: the listener understands, and objective knowledge appears transferred, only if he is prepared to understand.

HUMBERTO R. MATURANA,
BIOLOGY OF COGNITION

1
Acupuncture without Needles

TODAY, THE SCIENTIFIC RESULTS of years of research into Nutripuncture have broadened the medical world's view of the balance of the human body (female or male), its evolutionary course in connection with numerous environmental and historical parameters (the emotional family context in which a person grew up, the socio-cultural milieu in which a person was educated, a person's personal history, and so forth), and has been found to provide the necessary tools for the maturation of an individual's sensory and cognitive potential. This is most likely the reason why Edgar Morin describes this approach as "biological humanism."

Nutripuncture is fascinating in many areas, whether it involves supporting the body during crucial stages of growth, overcoming the difficult ordeals life sometimes sends our way, or dealing with stress. For example, it can enhance the performance of an athlete or augment the voice of a speaker or singer. It can improve coordination and motor skills in vital functions like walking. In osteopathy, it allows a more effective rehabilitation, especially at the postural and joint level. In odontology, the regulation of the vital currents reinforces the body's environment and thus allows better results at the level of dental care, periodontal surgeries, implants, and so forth.

Nutripuncture is not so much a therapy, however, as an approach that is capable of reinforcing the internal cellular "terrain," which can be disturbed by functional disorders, as well as biological and organic malfunctions. There are two types of terrains: one is innate, hereditary, passed on genetically; the other is acquired by the individual as the fruit of personal experiences and the particular way he or she behaves. Disease appears when a decline of the vital potential within a system weakens the terrain, making it vulnerable to dysfunction. Nutripuncture makes it possible to reinforce the vitality of the organism, protect its integrity, and promote well-being. It also enhances self-knowledge by awakening sensory and cognitive potential, which may often have failed to find expression. It accomplishes all this by restoring the flow of the vital currents, which—in acupuncture—are mapped by well-defined lines known as meridians.

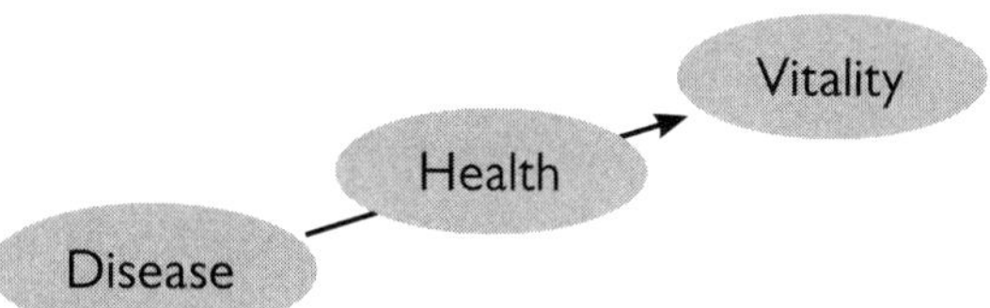

Fig. 1.1. The stronger our vitality, the further we move away from the instability of disease (the definition of *health* being "absence of disease").

In acupuncture theory, the meridians map the flow of information within the body and between the body and its environment, governing both internal and external communication, cooperation, and coordination of all aspects of the organism. To better grasp this theory—still foreign to our culture and often too complex to comprehend—it is important to understand the three concepts it is composed of: meridian, vital current, and information.

We can be aided in this by a familiar metaphor, an image that everyone knows: the subway. An intricate network of destinations and connections, it evokes the network of the meridian lines that circulate through the body.

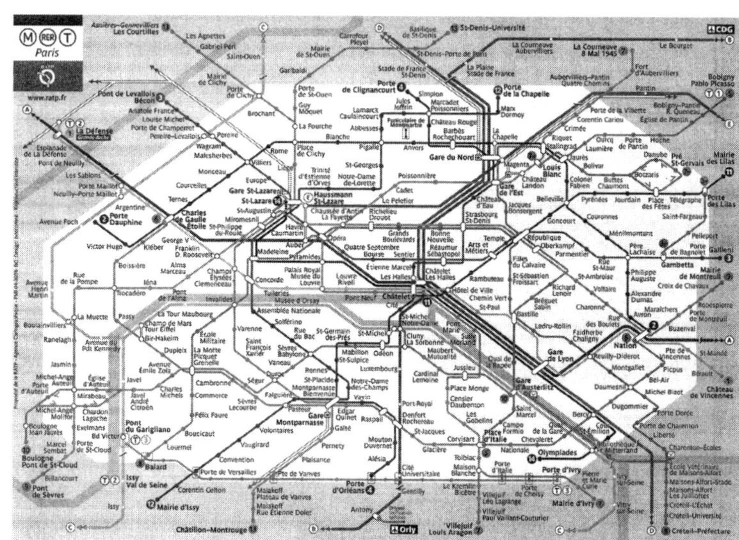

Fig. 1.2. Map of the Paris Metro

Lines = Meridians
Trains = Vital Currents
Passengers = Information

The Paris subway system, for example, is composed of several underground lines, each of which is numbered (1–14). Each line communicates with the others via transfer stations (such as Châtelet, Republic, Star). Similarly, the meridians communicate via energetic points. The vital currents (trains) circulate on the meridian lines, charged with environmental information (passengers). The vital currents are time sensitive, just like the subway trains that run according to schedules, which vary by the hour, day of the week, or period of the year.

Meridians and Subways Are Analogous

Meridian lines are constitutional layouts (like subway lines) found in humans.

Vital currents (like the trains) circulate the data.

Information (like the passengers), formed by stimuli received from the environment and from within, is transported along the lines.

WHAT ARE THE MERIDIANS?

The meridian lines are the vectors of environmental information necessary for proper modulation of organic and mental life. Although they are not directly responsible for any molecular reaction, they circulate the impulses necessary to initiate all biochemical reactions. They guarantee the stability of the constitutional and acquired terrain of every person. The electrical activity of the meridians stops at death: although the molecules are still present, the vital currents no longer feed the tissues of the body.

Traditional acupuncture describes twelve main meridian lines, named according to the main organs they pass through, and are connected in pairs corresponding to their specific functions.

Kidneys and the Bladder
Stomach and the Spleen-Pancreas
Liver and the Gall Bladder
Master of Heart and Triple Warmer
Lungs and Colon/Large Intestine
Heart and Small Intestine

In addition to the meridian lines mentioned above, acupuncture also describes other meridian groups known as "marvelous" [also known as the eight "extraor-

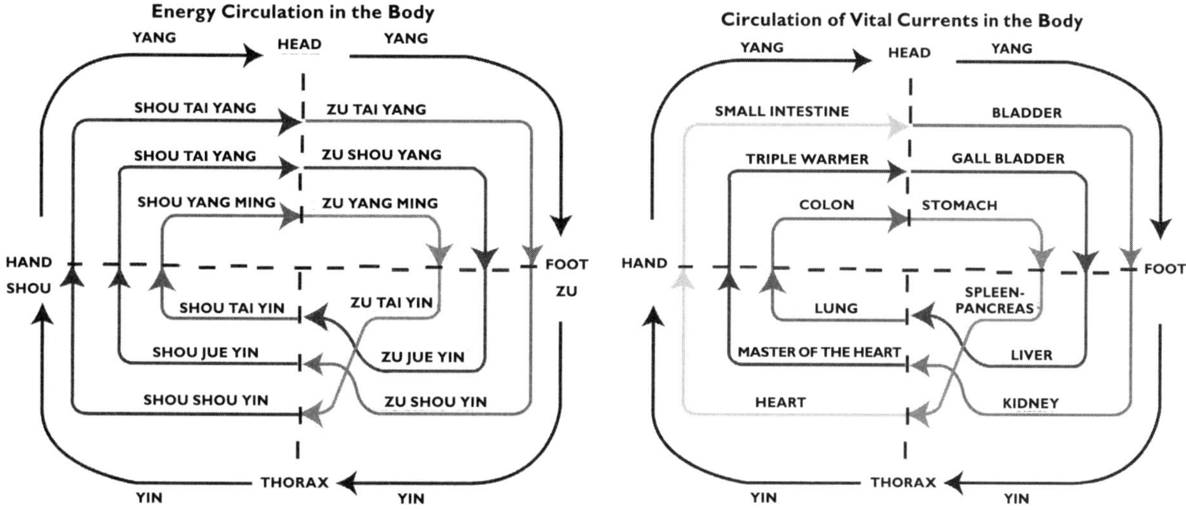

Fig 1.3. In the Eastern nomenclature each meridian line is named according to its pathway, beginning with the word *Shou* (if it starts on the upper limbs) or *Zu* (if it starts on the lower extremities).

dinary," "curious," or "irregular" vessels—*Trans.*], in particular the Conception Vessel and the Governor Vessel meridians.

In acupuncture, each meridian line is named according to the length of its pathway, its localization, and polarity (yin or yang). In the West, each line is named according to one of its functions. Thus the meridian line Shou Yang Ming, which circulates on the level of the upper limbs, is called Colon/Large Intestine. However, the role of each meridian is not limited to the function of the organs located along its route; rather it encompasses that of the various points it crosses on its way, thus ensuring global communication between every sector of the body. This is similar to the famous Route 66 that crosses the United States from Chicago, Illinois, to Santa Monica, California. Yes, the highway does go to the West Coast, but along the way it goes through other cities and communicates with them. The electromagnetic circuits of communication connecting various organs are composed of a succession of points located by measuring musculo-cutaneous resistance. They outline vital tension lines, corresponding to the morphogenetic currents set up since embryogenesis.

Nutripuncture uses fourteen primary meridian lines and twenty-four secondary lines (of which five are specifically female and five male), resulting in thirty-eight meridian lines in all. All of the Nutripuncture meridians systematically wend their way through the left and right parts of the body, except for the two central meridians, which travel along the middle of the torso. These are the Governor Vessel, in back, and the Conception Vessel, in front. (See color insert.)

The Fourteen Principal Nutripuncture Meridians Paired by Function

- The meridian line of the Heart with that of the Small Intestine
- The meridian line of the Lungs with that of the Colon
- The meridian line of the Stomach with that of the Spleen-Pancreas
- The meridian line of the Kidneys with that of the Bladder
- The meridian line of the Liver with that of the Gall Bladder
- The meridian line of the Master of the Heart with that of the Triple Warmer
- The meridian line of Conception with that of the Governor

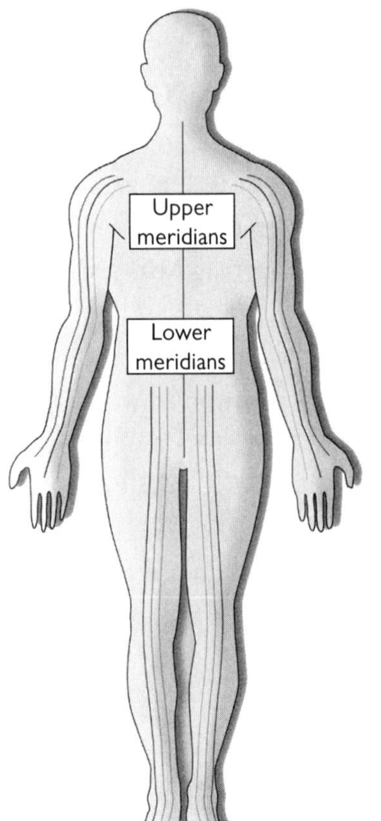

Fig. 1.4. The meridians of the body are divided into upper and lower.

The secondary meridian lines used in Nutripuncture were indexed and classified during recent research undertaken with human beings in modern settings. In today's society, humankind lives and interacts with a stimulus-rich environment, one that is very different from that during the era when the meridian lines in acupuncture were revealed, thousands of years ago. Similarly, continuing research in the field of traditional Chinese medicine is constantly revealing new acupuncture points with special functions. Additionally, Eastern teachings that were conceived in an imagistic language have been translated in the West to an organic language that combines images with purely physiological functions.

In Nutripuncture each meridian line is labeled by a number from 01 to 38. This enables us to extricate ourselves from the Western "physiological" vision, which has diverted the holistic spirit of acupuncture, and to recover an overall view of the vital currents and their functions. In the later chapters, we will therefore refer to the meridians by their numbers (although we will provide their correspondences with the official classification in the beginning) in order to provide a better idea of their function, which is often connected to their pathway. These pathways are not localized like an organ but are quite varied and highly complex. Each of the meridian lines and their functions will be described in detail in chapter 2.

UNDERSTANDING VITAL CURRENTS

The Nutripuncture research conducted on people of modern times takes into consideration their interaction with an environment that is greatly charged with stimuli and quite different from the context that witnessed the birth of acupuncture thousands of years ago. The last century has been witness to many revolutions and paradigm shifts (cultural, social, in human relationships and communications), which have necessarily been accompanied by profound changes in the body, in cellular communication, and cerebral organization. Thanks to its plasticity, the body has no doubt called for the activation of new vital currents in order to better manage the massive amounts of information that come from the interaction of billions of human beings with an environment that is evolving and producing at an amazing speed.

This is why, in contrast to acupuncture, Nutripuncture makes it possible to attack the behavioral disorders affecting humans today, which weaken the vitality of their vital currents and pave the way for new disorders. Its purpose is therefore to modulate the expression of an emotional, sensory, and cognitive potential, which is sorely tested by a lifestyle that is often incompatible with the body's natural rhythms and inhibits the expression of the elements of which it is made (Water, Air, Earth, Fire, and Ether) and which are also present in our planet.

JUST WHAT DO WE MEAN BY INFORMATION PRECISELY?

Everything in reality is information, everything carries an intrinsic message: a flower, a rainbow, a sound, an odor, a fruit, a landscape, a face, an animal, a tree, a drawing, a poem . . . everything has a meaning and stimulates our perception. A shape, a color, or a musical note has a presence, a particular message for our visual or auditory cells. The sensations emerging from this sensory contact are the source of what we know, which is not the same as what we learn in school, which is often purely cognitive information amputated from the sensual and sensory reality of the body.

Everything in our natural, social, and cultural environment is information. Every element, like every being, carries messages revealing its life impulse. The way we deal with information—how we integrate and respond to it—calls on the inner organization of each individual, our unique neurological organization that has been shaped by our experiences.

As Edgar Morin explains, "The human organism is a very elaborate system formed of different elements (which are antagonistic and complementary at the same time), whose cooperation forms a whole in which they preserve their distinct character. In the organic domain, the play of interactions calls on principles unknown to the world of chemistry, which is to say notions of information, codes, messages . . . concepts pulled from the experience of human relationships."[1]

As in a society, each organ plays an essential role in maintaining the life of the body, thanks to its unique and interactive function with the other systems. The meridians play a major role in the organic communication that ensures the circulation of the information necessary for cellular cooperation and self-regulation.

PSYCHOPHYSICAL VITALITY: A FRAGILE BALANCE THAT DEPENDS ON THE INTERACTION BETWEEN OUR CONTEXT AND OURSELVES

Life could not blossom and grow without the stimuli provided by our environment. These are the essential impulses we need to activate and maintain the vital functions, programmed in our genes, which encourage individual development. Gustatory, auditory, olfactory, visual, and tactile stimuli travel through our sensory receptors, whose performance level is responsible for the harmonious perception of reality in all its forms, colors, smells, sounds, and flavors. They also enable us to communicate with our personal context, with our fellow humans, and all other life forms. Although perception is an entirely individual matter, the overall integrated perception of reality depends on the circulation of the vital currents that feed our sensory receptors: the mouth, ears, nose, eyes, and skin.

While stimuli are necessary for the emergence and budding of the dormant personality within each of us, they also can, if they are insufficient or in excess, induce a whole variety of physical or psychological disturbances. The absence of a stimulus causes regression of its related function. For example: without sound and vocal stimuli, a newborn will not be able to learn the native language; without light stimuli, laboratory animals would go blind; the immobility caused by wearing a cast induces joint stiffness and muscular mass depletion. Alternatively, excessive stimuli can induce stress that can trigger defense mechanisms and disturb the balance of certain organ functions.

By empiric use of different mineral complexes, Nutripuncture research has made it possible to list the impact of various kinds of stress on the balance of the vital currents, which are always adaptable to the reactive and adaptive capacities of the individual.

THE TOOLS OF NUTRIPUNCTURE: THE NUTRIS

In contrast to acupuncture treatment performed with needles, in Nutripuncture the optimal dynamics of the thirty-eight meridians are encouraged by thirty-eight Nutris. In addition Nutripuncture uses one more Nutri, the General Cellular Nutritional Regulator known as Nutri Yin–Nutri Yang, which regulates cell communication. Aside from Nutri Yin–Nutri Yang, each Nutri has a number, target, and a function, corresponding with the Nutripuncture meridians.

The focus of Nutripuncture is on restoring vital currents and not acting against symptoms and disease. The self-regulation of the organism is impaired when the vital currents are not in balance. Both Nutripuncture and acupuncture work to regulate the electromagnetic circulation of the meridians, but in acupuncture activation of the meridians varies in relation to the actions of the therapist. The Nutris, on the other hand, are precise and activate the meridians exactly the same way in every person, which gives an unparalleled consistency.

Each Nutri is a unique and precise synergistic combination of trace minerals whose function is to activate each meridian. Just as a perfect chocolate cream pastry results from the art of baking and mixing ingredients, the Nutris result from the art of mixing trace minerals to restore the vital currents. For the pastry, the ingredients—chocolate, egg whites, sugar, milk, and so on—have to be properly combined. Salt can't be substituted for sugar, nor butter for milk. If the ingredients are not mixed in the proper order, the pastry will not come out well. If there is any slight variation in the construction of the Nutris, they *will not* properly activate the vital currents.

The perfected Nutri recipes are preserved in pills composed of neutralized lactose, sorbitol, and magnesium stearate (emulsifier). The lactose is an essential ingredient, which enhances the action of the trace minerals. Two ranges of lactose are used; when they are combined with sorbitol, the allergenic effects of lactose are neutralized. This is significant because it makes the Nutris compatible for *all* people. The Nutris have a very pleasant, mildly sweet taste. Because of their pleasant taste they are agreeable to everyone and easy to administer to children. The Nutris are manufactured in a French factory by Laboratoires Pronutri and classified as a nutritional supplement by the FDA.

The information preserved in the Nutris is activated immediately upon chewing. Because the cellular memory is very strong and deep, the information must be restored consistently to rewire the meridian network. Usually the Nutris are taken twice a day for one month, but this can vary depending on the level of disturbance. Because each Nutri pill activates specific information for its related meridian, each pill must be chewed and swallowed completely before the next one is chewed.

39 Nutris Working for Our Vitality

Nutri 01 • meridian line 01—the gift, vital currents of the Arteries

Nutri 02 • meridian line 02—postural balance, vital currents of the Cerebellum

Nutri 03 • meridian line 03—potency, vital currents of the Hair

Nutri 04 • meridian line 04—rhythm and decision, vital currents of the Heart

Nutri 05 • meridian line 05—organization, vital currents of the Colon

Nutri 06 • meridian line 06—male sexuality, vital currents the Penis

Nutri 07 • meridian line 07—female sexuality, vital currents of the Vagina

Nutri 08 • meridian line 08—cognitive integration, vital currents of the Cerebral Cortex

Nutri 09 • meridian line 09—source energy, vital currents of the Adrenal Glands

Nutri 10 • meridian line 10—action, vital currents of the Stomach

Nutri 11 • meridian line 11—metabolic activation, vital currents of the Liver

Nutri 12 • meridian line 12—instinct, vital currents of the Hypothalamus

Nutri 13 • meridian line 13—choice, vital currents of the Small Intestine

Nutri 14 • meridian line 14—virility, vital currents of the Adam's Apple

Nutri 15 • meridian line 15—self-expression, vital currents of the Lymphatic Glands

Nutri 16 • meridian line 16—movement, vital currents of the Muscles

Nutri 17 • meridian line 17—structure, vital currents of the Bones

Nutri 18 • meridian line 18—transformation, vital currents of the Pancreas

Nutri 19 • meridian line 19—tactility, vital currents of the Skin

Nutri 20 • meridian line 20—the breath, vital currents of the Lungs

Nutri 21 • meridian line 21—anchoring and male realization, the vital currents of the Prostate

Nutri 22 • meridian line 22—assurance, vital currents of the Kidneys

Nutri 23 • meridian line 23—representation, vital currents of the Retina

Nutri 24 • meridian line 24—femininity, vital currents of the Breasts

Nutri 25 • meridian line 25—inspiration, vital currents of the Sinus

Nutri 26 • meridian line 26—motor conduction, vital currents of the Thalamus

Nutri 27 • meridian line 27—time, vital currents of the Thyroid

Nutri 28 • meridian line 28—female anchoring and realization, vital currents of the Uterus

Nutri 29 • meridian line 29—receptivity, vital currents of the Veins

Nutri 30 • meridian line 30—metabolic regulation, vital currents of the Gallbladder

Nutri 31 • meridian line 31—vigilance, vital currents of the Bladder

Nutri 32 • meridian line 32—vision, vital currents of Sight

Nutri 33 • meridian line 33—spatial orientation, vital currents of Conception

Nutri 34 • meridian line 34—spatial orientation, vital currents of the Governor

Nutri 35 • meridian line 35—female cerebral activation, vital currents of the Master of the Heart

Nutri 36 • meridian line 36—male cerebral activation, vital currents of the Master of the Heart

Nutri 37 • meridian line 37—female cerebral regulation, vital currents of the Triple Warmer

Nutri 38 • meridian line 38—male cerebral regulation, vital currents of the Triple Warmer

Nutri Yin–Nutri Yang—general regulation of cellular communication

NUTRIPUNCTURE APPLICATIONS

Empirical research has made it possible to develop many interesting protocols based on the application of these Nutris. In particular, two primary modes of application have been found to be very effective, which we have labeled Associative Nutripuncture and Sequential Nutripuncture.

Associative Nutripuncture

Associative Nutripuncture is used to stimulate the potential and self-regulation of weakened meridian lines. In this application the General Cellular Nutritional Regulator is combined with Nutris corresponding to meridians showing need of regulation. For example, the meridians of the Kidneys (22) and the Bladder (31) are particularly sensitive during the winter season. So Associative Nutripuncture would suggest the use of the General Cellular Nutritional Regulator plus Nutri 22 and Nutri 31 during the winter to reinforce these circuits. This combination is also therapeutic in the event of timidity, fear, or lack of assurance, and so on, which are all emotions related to those organs. This application of Nutripuncture is described in detail in part 2 of the book.

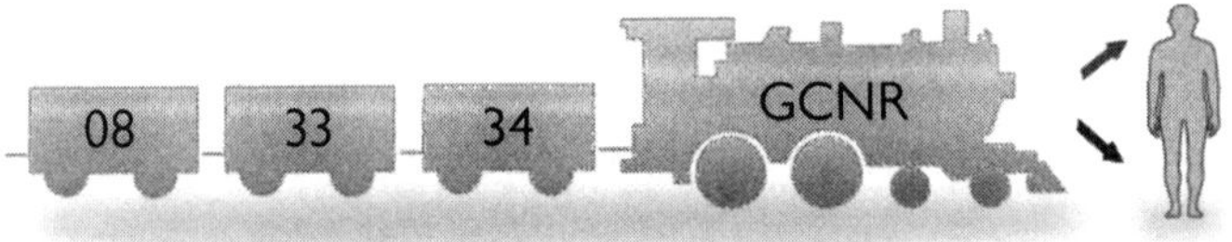

Fig. 1.5. In Associative Nutripuncture, the General Cellular Nutritional Regulator plays the role of a locomotive for each Nutri and its corresponding meridian.

Sequential Nutripuncture

Sequential Nutripuncture is more complex than Associative Nutripuncture, as it is related to specific aspects of the individual's development and exposure and the impact on the organism. Ongoing Nutripuncture research over the past twenty years has studied the impact of a large number of stress inducers on the vital currents of the body. In fact, each kind of stress weakens the body's vitality and inhibits the sensitivity of one of the five senses, depending on the individual's particular perception. As a result, the psychophysical consequences of stress can be quite different from one individual to the next, although the body always uses the same circuits when reacting to one kind of stress. For example, whenever a person is dealing with work-related stress (action potential), the same vital currents are always involved: the Stomach, the Pancreas, and the Uterus (or the Prostate for men).

Thanks to the clinical experience of many practitioners, many different protocols have been perfected to regulate the meridians that have been rendered most fragile by tragic events such as a mourned loss, divorce, abortion, rape, and so on. Use of these protocols has demonstrated that the stimulation of the vital currents encouraged an optimal psychophysical dynamic, allowing the individual to recognize the impact of stress on his or her equilibrium, and how to "digest" it in order to overcome it and grow. Each of life's experiences then becomes the means for attaining the fullness of the human dimension.

In addition, experiments conducted in several fields have investigated the elements necessary for the awakening of an individual's genetic potential as well as the emotional and cognitive maturation of the balanced human. Thanks to the clinical observation of many experts, this research today constitutes invaluable material for better integrating the complexity of the organism with its individual psychophysical expression, which is in constant interaction with its natural and social environment. Sequential Nutripuncture offers a general reorganization of the ground in the body while regulating, stage after stage, the circuits that were not sufficiently stimulated during the learning process.

For example, the "Oedipus complex," recognized as one of the fundamental stages of individual self-recognition as a sexual being, permits each child to find his or her place in relation to the opposite sex and represents the first step in training for future social life interactions. Thanks to research trials run by multiple practitioners, it has been observed that when this stage is experienced inadequately or poorly integrated at the cognitive level, it can result in some behavioral and functional troubles during adulthood, connected with an insufficient flow in certain meridian lines. For more efficient assimilation of this period, or to solve its aftereffects during adulthood, specific sequences of five Nutris are used to regulate the circuits concerned.

In part 3 of this book, this and several other of the specific ways of using Sequential Nutripuncture are introduced.

Seasonal Nutripuncture

In addition to these two primary applications, other approaches have been developed as well. One simple way to approach Nutripuncture and appreciate its benefits is to use it in accordance with the seasons. This means focusing on specific vital currents seasonally, as the different meridians are more sensitive at certain times of the year. This approach is presented in detail in chapter 5, "Maintaining Vitality through Every Season of the Year."

2
The Meridians and Us

THE PAIRINGS of the principal meridians are based on three factors:

Anatomical pathway (related to the upper or lower limbs)
Rhythmic activity (which is more intense at certain hours)
Hierarchical organization (connected with function)

Four of the principal meridian pairs are associated with the target organs they encounter on their course: the Heart/Small Intestine, the Stomach/Spleen-Pancreas, the Lungs/Colon, the Kidneys/Bladder, and the Liver/Gall Bladder. The other two pairs, Master of the Heart/Triple Warmer, and Governor/Conception, do not encounter any of the key organs on their route, but have a unique functional nature. Unlike the others, the activity of the Governor Vessel and the Conception Vessel is not rhythmic but constant and temporally stable.

The meridian lines most connected with metabolic functioning are considered to be located in the lower limbs, even though their routes travel throughout the body; they are governed by the Liver/Gall Bladder pair, which also form the preeminent center for blood regulation in the body.

The upper extremities house the more rhythmic or neural meridian lines, which have an extra-sensitive and projective role; they are controlled by the Master of the Heart/Triple Warmer pair, which, with the Cerebral Cortex, form the pole regulating nerve activity.

The different types of meridians—metabolic and rhythmic/neural—form families to which the secondary meridians are attached. For example, the Kidneys/

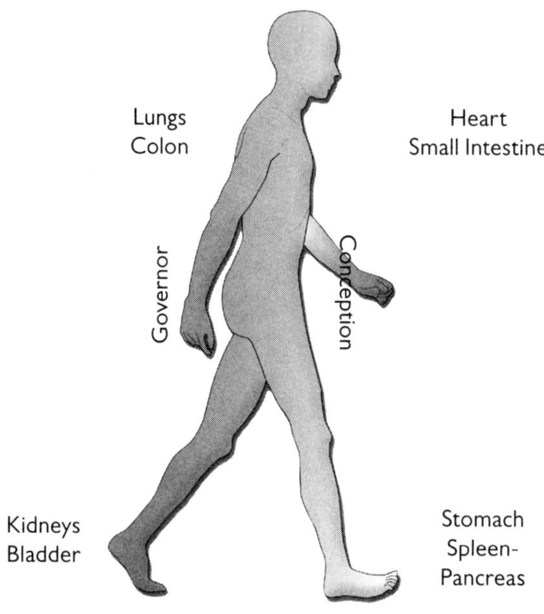

Fig. 2.1. Rhythmic or neural meridians are associated with the upper limbs of the body; metabolic meridians are associated with the lower limbs of the body.

Bladder family includes the meridian lines of the Adrenal Glands, the Cerebellum, and the Thyroid, among others (the secondary meridians of each family will be described in chapters seven and eight).

In the following depictions of the meridians, we are giving you a glimpse of the meridians' superficial course, although they also possess much deeper networks. Although the meridian lines are shown in the figures only on one side of the body, each of the meridians symmetrically traverses both sides of the body, with the exception of the Conception Vessel and Governor Vessel, which flow through the center of the body.

THE METABOLIC MERIDIANS OF THE LOWER HALF OF THE BODY (LOWER LIMBS)

These first three meridian pairs especially regulate activities of a metabolic nature. They carry information of a genetic and therefore innate nature and play a major role from conception to puberty. They regulate the circulation of the information necessary for fetal life, from physical growth to placement in life, and assure the gradual awakening of the cerebral pole and the neural/rhythm meridians. In adulthood they ensure the energy necessary for metabolism and the constant changes of the body.

Kidneys/Bladder (22/31) Family

The activity of this family regulates the circulation of the information contained in the genetic program and shapes the expression of a person's original code: his or her DNA. The joint activity of meridians 22 (Liver) and 31 (Bladder) also controls the exchange of information connected with the sexual codes (XX or XY). They regulate all fluid exchange and the metabolizing of carbohydrates. Meridian line 31 has particular points on its dorsal route that are called *mirrors* because they reflect the dynamics of the other meridians. Because of their complex route, these meridians are regarded as extremely vigilant sentinels that monitor the vitality of every sector of the body.

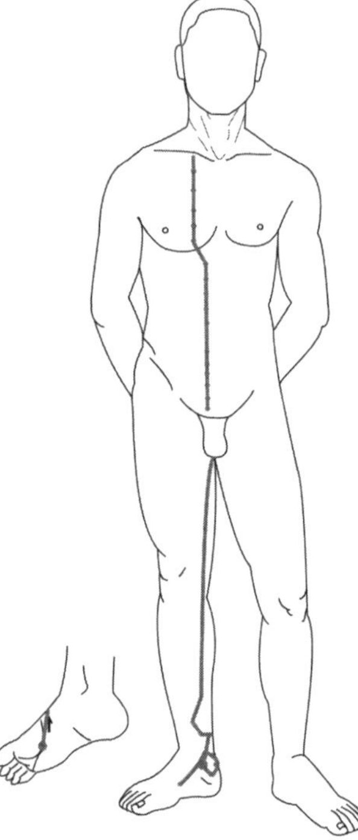

Fig. 2.2 (left). Pathway of Kidney Meridian Line 22

Meridian line 22 of the kidneys starts at the sole of each foot, travels up the inner legs and thighs, then through the abdomen and rib cage, and ends at the lower edge of the shoulder blades.

Fig. 2.3 (right). Pathway of Bladder Meridian Line 31

Meridian line 31 of the Bladder has a fairly long and complex course. It begins at the inner part of the eye, climbs toward the forehead to wend its way over the skull, then descends to the nape of the neck and the back, where it divides into two vertical branches, parallel to the spine, which then cross through the buttocks, wend their way over the back surface of the thighs and calves and come to an end in the little toe (outer edge).

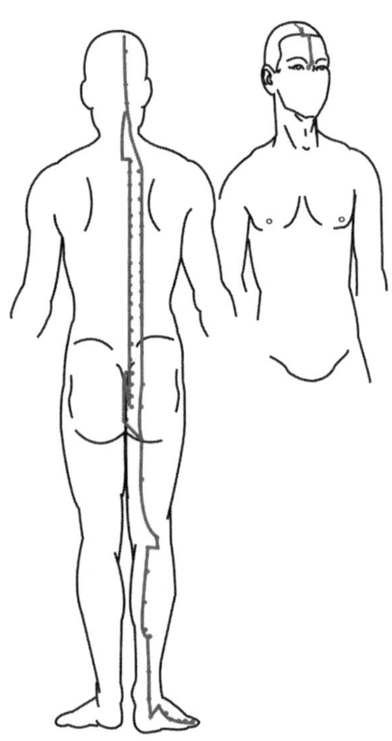

Stomach/Spleen-Pancreas (10/18) Family

The growth of the body is governed by meridians 10 (Stomach) and 18 (Spleen-Pancreas), which generate the activity necessary to build and transform tissue. This family of meridians watches over the balance of general protein metabolism and the skeletal frame in particular.

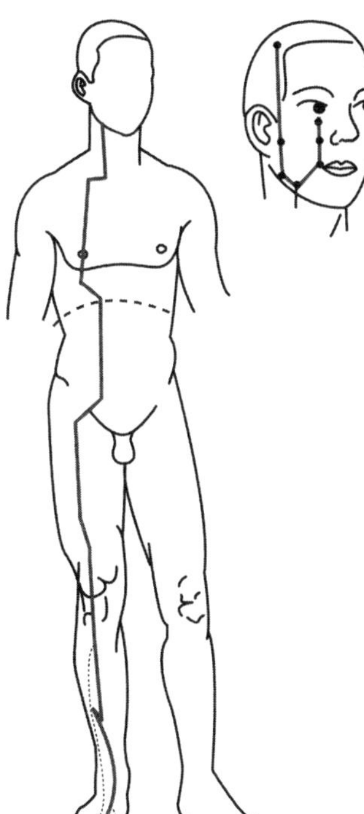

Fig. 2.4 (left). Pathway of the Stomach Meridian Line 10

The meridian line 10 of the Stomach starts at the lower eyelids, travels down the cheeks and jaw, the throat, rib cage, and abdomen before wending its way over the anterolateral surfaces of the thighs and legs, and coming to an end on the second toe of both feet.

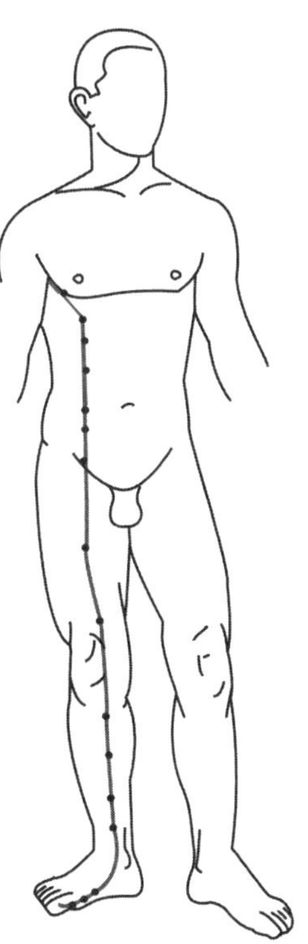

Fig. 2.5 (right). Pathway of the Pancreas Meridian Line 18

The meridian line 18 of the Pancreas starts in the middle of the big toes, wends its way over the inner surfaces of the legs and thighs before climbing through the abdomen and ribcage. Its course ends beneath the armpits, in the sixth intercostals space.

Liver/Gallbladder (11/30) Family: The Metabolic Pole

Meridian lines 11 (Liver) and 30 (Gall Bladder), shown on page 26, play a major role in the adjustment of the body's metabolic drive, generated by the joint activity of the families 22/31 and 10/18. This family is thus the pole of metabolic blood regulation. It also represents the nourishing center of the body, where it plays a starring role during fetal life, regulating the blood bond between mother and embryo. The Gall Bladder and Spleen meridians play a major role in blood dynamics. The activity of this family is complementary to that of the cerebral neural center (meridians of the upper half of the body: 35/37 for women and 36/38 for men). Their harmonious interaction ensures optimal self-regulation of the metabolism and nervous system.

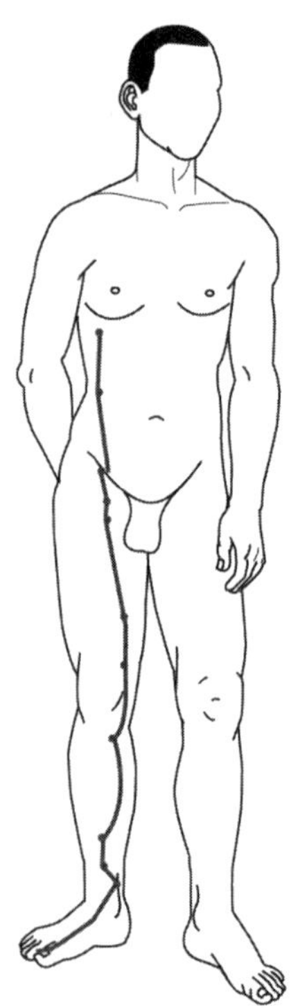

Fig. 2.6 (left). Pathway of the Liver Meridian Line 11

Meridian line 11 of the liver starts its course over the big toes of both feet, ascends up the inner legs and middle of the thighs directed toward the genital region. It then crosses through the stomach before entering the liver. It continues its route toward the rib cage and ends in the sixth intercostals space.

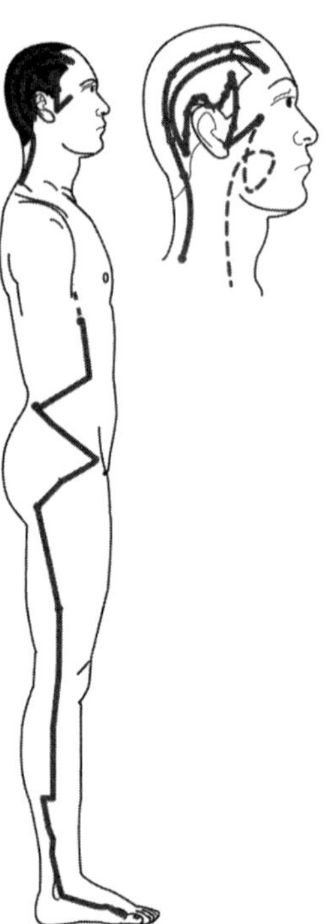

Fig. 2.7 (right). Pathway of the Gall Bladder Meridian Line 30

The meridian line 30 of the Gall Bladder starts at the outer corner of the eyelids and travels toward the ears, then climbs toward the temporal fossa where it makes three arcs before descending toward the nape and shoulders. It then travels down the lateral surfaces of the torso, hips, thighs, and legs. It descends to the feet, passing in front of the outer malleolus before coming to an end at the fourth toe. It is among the longest and most complex meridian lines of the entire network.

THE NEURAL/RHYTHM MERIDIANS OF THE UPPER HALF OF THE BODY (UPPER LIMBS)

In the course of individual growth and development, these meridians awaken gradually, thanks to the metabolic activity of the meridians of the lower half of the body. They play a starring role in adolescence and adulthood. In contrast to the meridians of the body's lower extremities, the nerve currents shape the circulation of acquired information, gained from personal experiences, which shapes individual personality and encourages cognitive maturation.

Lungs/Colon (20/05) Family

This family becomes completely functional at puberty, making it possible for individual sexual expression. This appears through a polarization of the upper half of the body (appearance of secondary sexual characteristics such as breasts and Adam's apple), triggered by the hormonal concert conducted by the secondary meridians of the Hypothalamus and Gonads, in accordance with the gender (XX or XY) manifested at birth. For their action of hormonal balance and emotional equilibrium, these meridians play a major role in the building of sexual identity. They also shape the vitality of the body's natural defenses, the acid-alkaline balance (pH-rH2) and air exchanges in general.

With the Kidneys/Bladder (22/31) family, these meridians form the central reference frame for body communication and air and fluid exchanges.

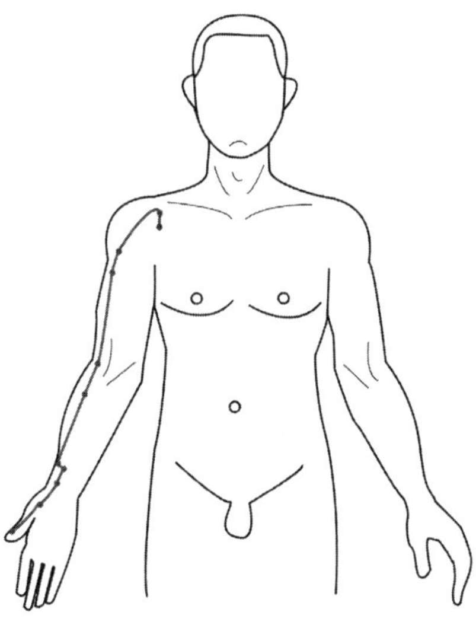

Fig. 2.8 (left). Pathway of Lungs Meridian Line 20

Meridian line 20 of the Lungs starts in the ribcage at the level of the first intercostal space. It then descends along the inner edges of the biceps toward the elbows, forearms, and wrists before ending in the tips of the thumbs.

Fig. 2.9 (right). Pathway of Colon Meridian Line 05

The meridian line 05 of the Colon starts in the tips of the index fingers and climbs toward the wrists from where it travels along the posterolateral surfaces of the forearms and arms up to the shoulders. It then wends its way over the lateral edges of the neck, climbs up the cheeks, winding around the upper lip before the two parts intersect and end at the nasal wings.

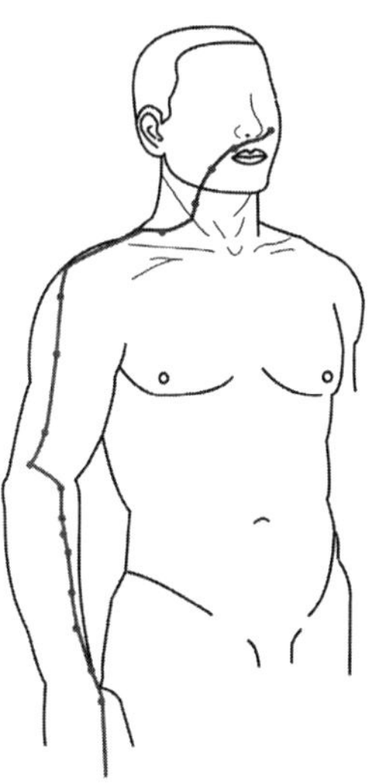

Heart/Small Intestine (04/13) Family

This family becomes completely functional at adulthood, making it possible for the human being to achieve cognitive maturity, self-awareness, and environmental awareness. Meridians 04 (Heart) and 13 (Small Intestine), shown on page 28, regulate circulatory balance, selective assimilation of foods, and the metabolizing of lipids. They also adjust emotional balance, transporting the desire "to be" and to project oneself into life, to make choices guided by the Heart (04) and the Cerebral Cortex (08).

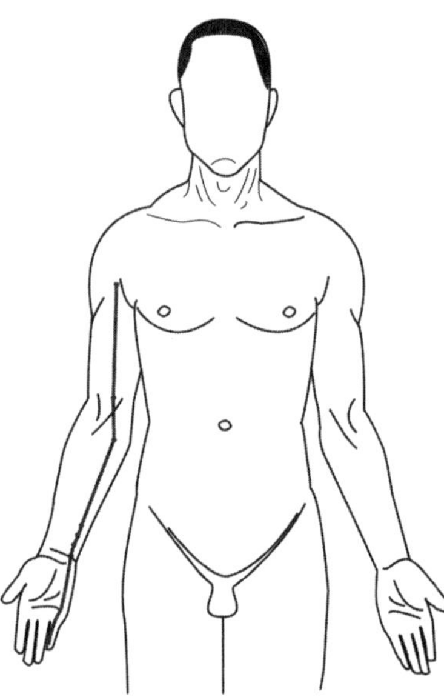

Fig. 2.10 (left). Pathway of the Heart Meridian Line 04

The meridian line 04 of the Heart starts in the center of the armpits, follows the inner edges of the anterior surface of the arms down to the elbows and forearms, then travels along the palms to end at the level of the little finger.

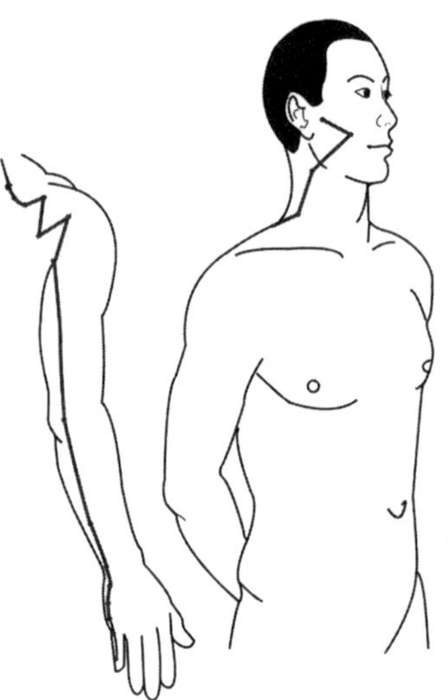

Fig. 2.11 (right). Pathway of the Small Intestine Meridian Line 13

The meridian line 13 of the Small Intestine starts at the corner of the little fingernail and follows the edge of the hand to the wrist. It continues to ascend along the posterior part of the arm up to the back of the shoulder joint. Internally, the line connects with the heart, and then travels in the direction of the esophagus, diaphragm, and stomach before entering the small intestine. Meanwhile, the external branch continues to travel up behind the muscle on the side of the neck and then over the cheek to the ear.

Master of the Heart/Triple Warmer (35/36 & 37/38) Family: Cerebral Pole

The Master of the Heart (35/36) and Triple Warmer (37/38) meridians are differently numbered for females and males. These meridians define space, form, and boundaries; they also contain the metabolic expansion of the Liver/Gall Bladder pair (11/30).

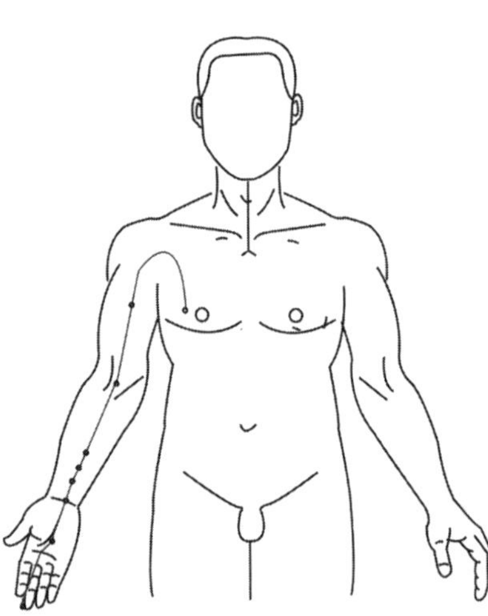

Fig. 2.12 (left). Pathway of the Master of the Heart Meridian Lines 35/36

The meridian lines 35/36 (female/male) of the Master of the Heart begin on the chest just outside the nipples, then descend along the anterior surfaces of the arms to the middle of the wrists. They then traverse the palms before coming to an end at the outer corner of the middle finger.

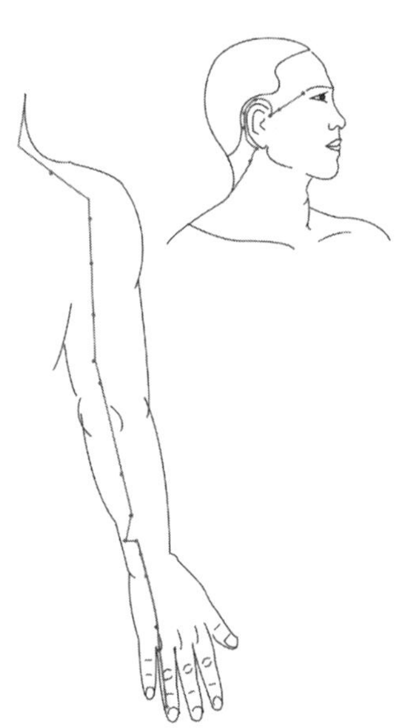

Fig. 2.13 (right). Pathway of the Triple Warmer Meridian Lines 37/38

The meridians 37/38 (female/male) of the Triple Warmer begin at each ring finger, wend their way along the outer edge of the arms to the shoulders and up the neck, continue traveling over the head, following the tops of the ears, and come to an end at the outer tips of the eyebrows.

Circulation of Vital Currents in the Body

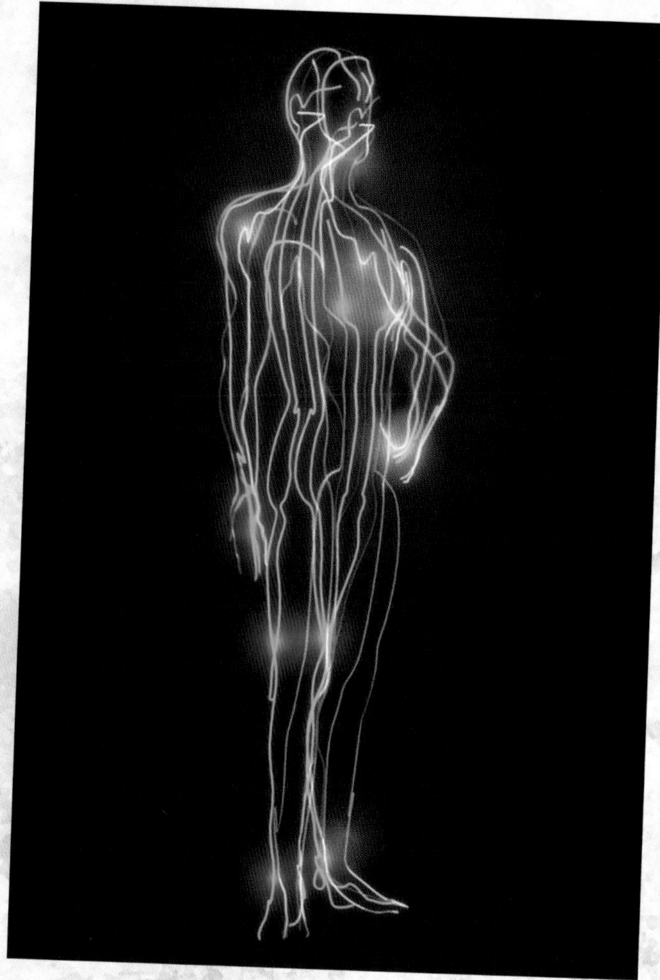

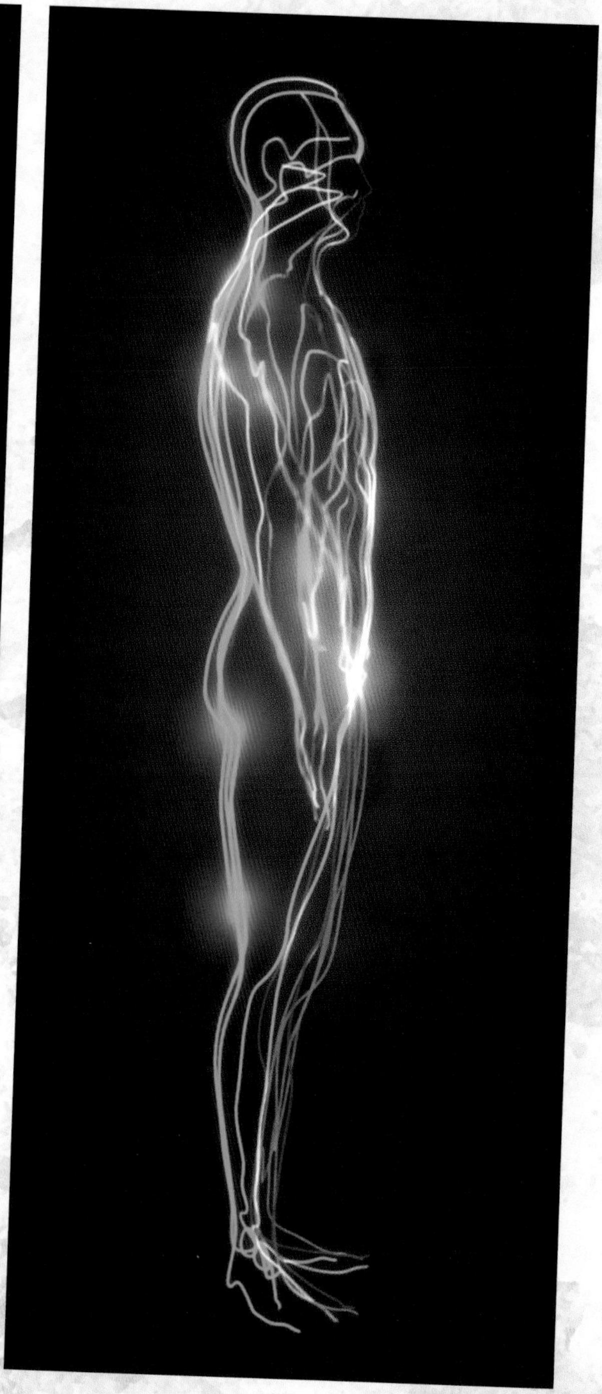

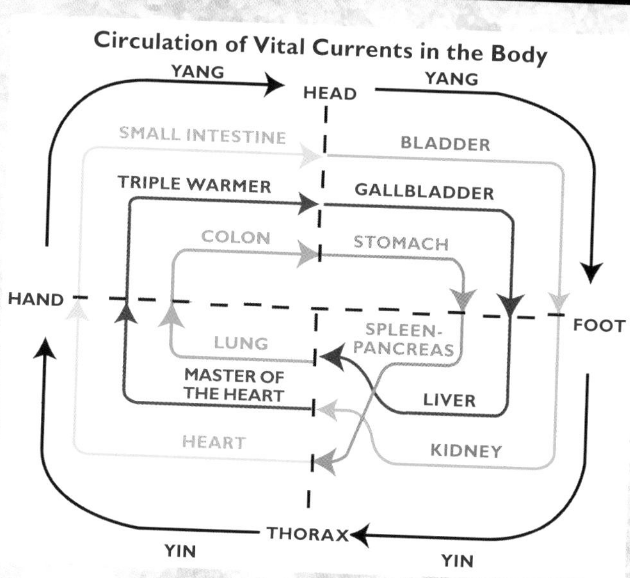

Nutripuncture uses 14 primary meridian lines and 24 secondary lines (38 meridian lines in total) in connection with the 5 senses and the 5 elements (Earth, Water, Air, Fire, and Ether). (See pages 12–15.)

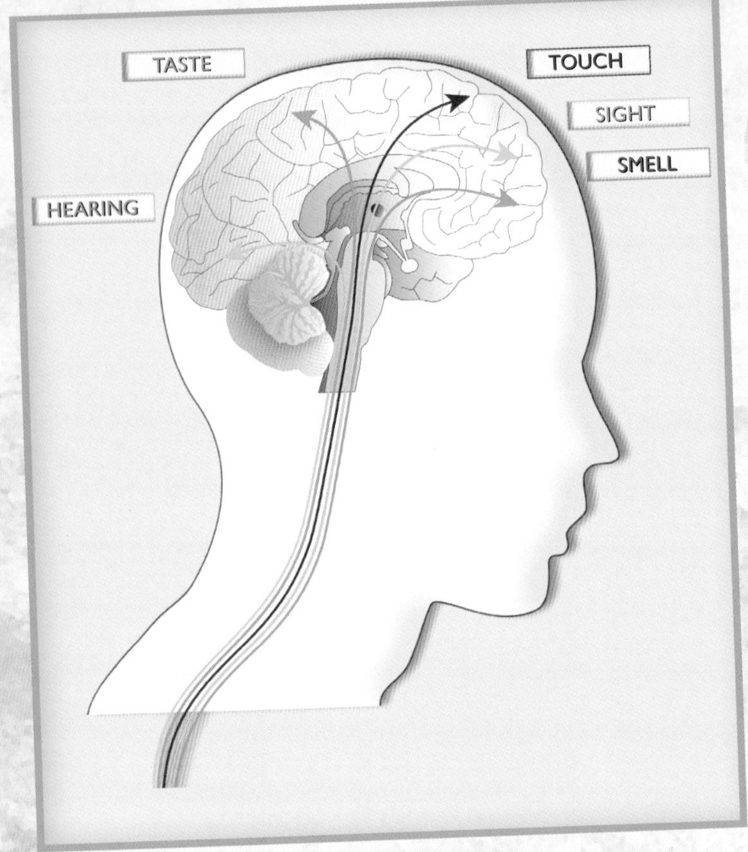

(Left) Our senses and, thus, the way we experience the world, are key factors in identity. (See pages 57–59.)

(Below left) Circadian rhythm of the meridians (see pages 47–48)

3:00 a.m. to 5:00 a.m. Lung meridian line 20 (Shou Tai Yin)

5:00 a.m. to 7:00 a.m. Colon meridian line 05 (Shou Yang Ming)

7:00 a.m. to 9:00 a.m. Stomach meridian line 10 (Zu Yang Ming)

9:00 a.m. to 11:00 a.m. Spleen-Pancreas meridian line 18 (Zu Tai Yin)

11:00 a.m. to 1:00 p.m. Heart meridian line 04 (Shou Shao Yin)

1:00 p.m. to 3:00 p.m. Small Intestine meridian line 13 (Shou Tai Yang)

3:00 p.m. to 5:00 p.m. Bladder meridian line 31 (Zu Tai Yang)

5:00 p.m. to 7:00 p.m. Kidney meridian line 22 (Zu Shao Yin)

7:00 p.m. to 9:00 p.m. Master of the Heart meridian lines 35/36 (Shou Jue Yin)

9:00 p.m. to 11:00 p.m. Triple Warmer meridian lines 37/38 (Shou Shao Yang)

11:00 p.m. to 1:00 a.m. Gall Bladder meridian line 30 (Zu Shao Yang)

1:00 a.m. to 3:00 a.m. Liver meridian line 11 (Zu Jue Yin)

They form the cerebral nerve center, which is complementary to the metabolic blood center. Their harmonious interaction ensures our optimal psychophysical dynamic. The Triple Warmer meridians, in particular, in synergy with the metabolic meridians 30 and 18, regulate the excess of the blood center.

The primary role of the Master of the Heart/Triple Warmer family is to adjust the activity of the meridians 20 and 05 and 04 and 13, and to polarize all the other meridians in their gender functions. This family therefore carries different information for women than it does for men.

THE CENTRAL MERIDIANS: CONCEPTION VESSEL AND GOVERNOR VESSEL (33/34)

This pair of meridians, called "primordial," appears very early during intrauterine life, tracing the axis of the embryo's development between the cerebral and the caudal poles, following the blueprint of the gene "architects." Their median pathway is essential because it connects the top and bottom parts of the body, separates right from left, and governs bipedal posture and human verticality.

These meridians are not connected to organs but—like the previous Master of

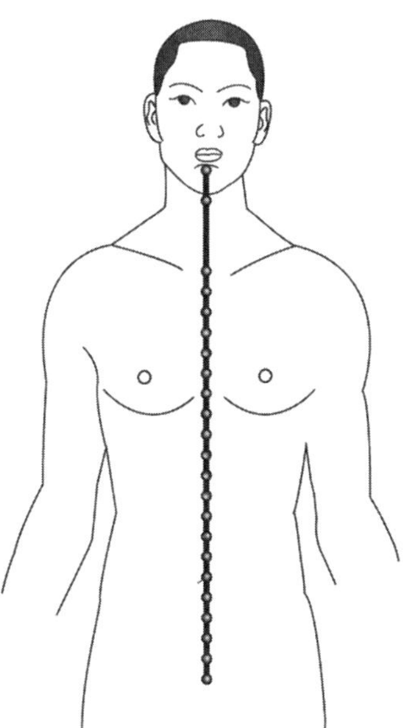

Fig. 2.14 (left). Median Pathway of the Conception Meridian 33

Meridian 33 of Conception starts in the perineum, climbs up the front surface of the body to the waist, crosses through the navel, sternum, throat, and jaw, and finishes its course at the level of the lower incisors.

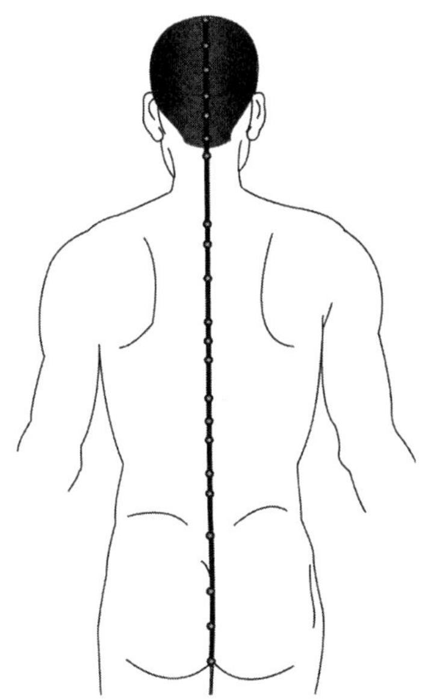

Fig. 2.15 (right). Median Pathway of the Governor Meridian 34

Meridian 34 of Governor starts in the perineum, climbs up the back surface of the body following the spinal column up through the back of the neck and head, and then comes back down the face over the forehead and along the nose to terminate at the level of the upper incisors.

the Heart and Triple Warmer pair—they regulate a fundamental function: spatial orientation, guarantee of harmonious growth, and balanced posture. They provide a major structural parameter around which every child organizes his or her body diagram while learning to move and walk. As the spinal column forms our structural axis, the Governor and Conception Meridians form the energetic axis of the body. Their circulation can often be disrupted and this has an influence over our verticality, both physical and mental. When these meridians are weakened, all the elements of the skeleton can be affected (spinal column, joints, dental occlusion, and so on). The individual can also exhibit numerous behavioral disorders and mental attitude can be disoriented and "out of it."

THE MERIDIANS: A DYNAMIC ORGANIZATION

If the construction of the body is ensured from conception to puberty by the impulse-driven activity of the metabolic meridians (stimulating the gradual awakening of the neural center), then the cerebral center will be able to launch into its role as the body's control tower during adulthood. It is this function that contains the metabolic impulse and regulates the individual's behavioral dynamic.

Adult behavior is the reflection of the principal meridians that are activated hierarchically but interdependently during the crucial stages of life: conception, birth, childhood, adolescence, and adulthood. The way these vital currents are shaped by the individual's experience—whether it is stimulating or stressful—will determine how they interact. Will they work together harmoniously or be out of order? In chapter 4 we will examine the impact of meridians on our behavior in greater detail. In the meantime here is a very succinct glimpse of their role in human developmental dynamics.

Before and After Birth: Every individual's capabilities are programmed by his or her genetic baggage (information shaped by the Kidneys/Bladder meridians) throughout intrauterine life. Concrete action undertaken following birth (governed by the Stomach/Spleen-Pancreas meridians) and all external stimuli, will allow the individual to unfold this potential and place its imprint deep in memory (fig. 2.16).

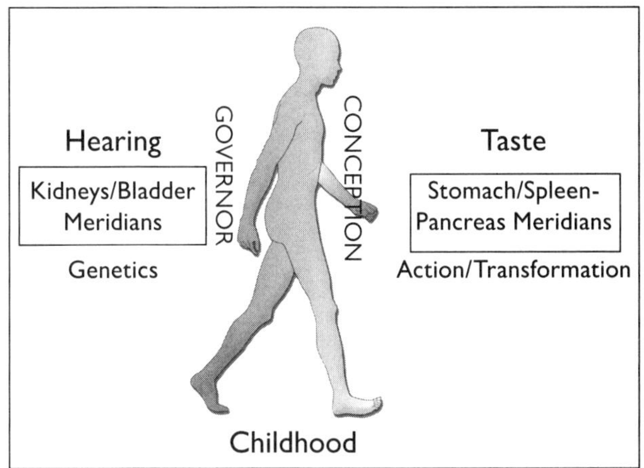

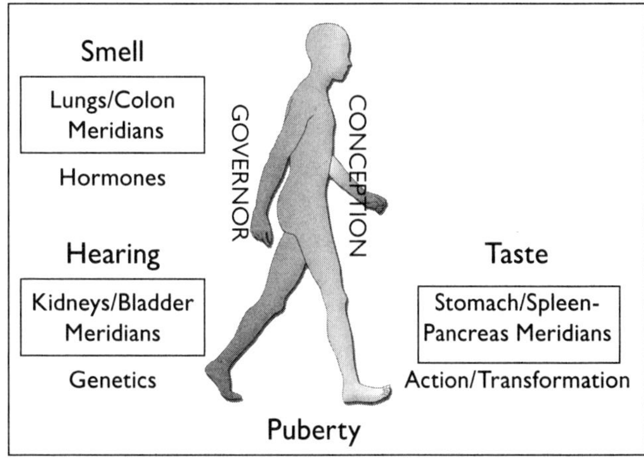

Fig. 2.16 (above). The activity of the lower body meridians ensures metabolic impulse and plays an essential role in the period from conception to puberty.

Fig. 2.17 (above right). The activity of the rhythmic meridians increases at puberty.

Fig. 2.18 (right). The activity of the projective meridians encourages adult cognitive maturity.

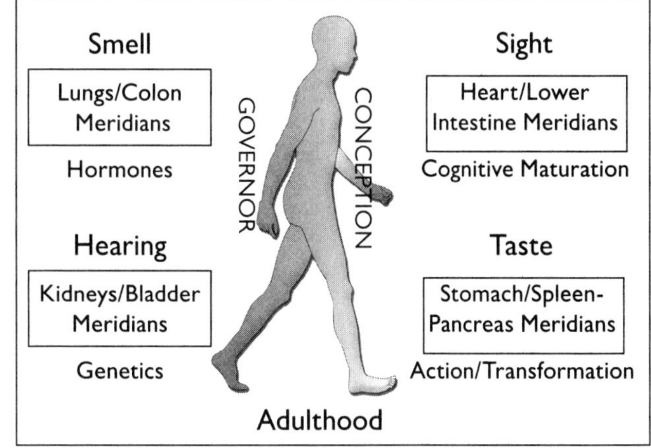

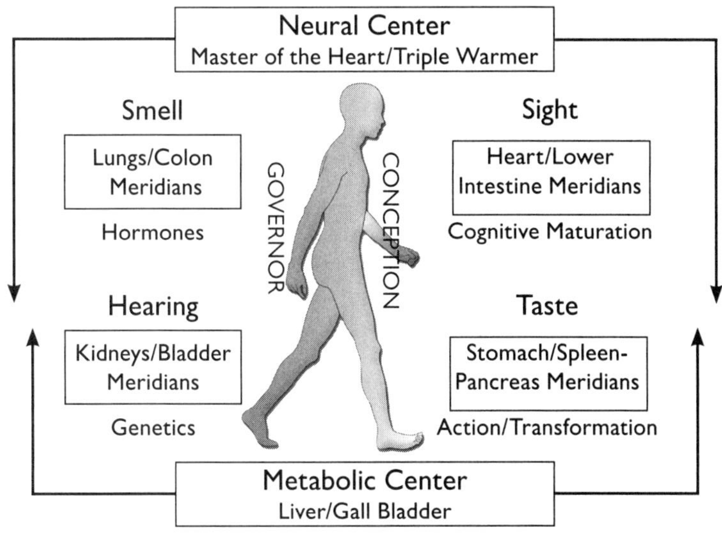

Fig. 2.19. Global dynamic of the meridians nourished by the metabolic center and contained by the neural center

Puberty: The activity of the Lungs/Colon meridians in puberty gives rhythm to the hormonal storms that trigger the changes of adolescence (fig. 2.17).

Adulthood: Adult cognitive maturation is ensured by the projective activity of the Heart/Small Intestine meridians (fig. 2.18).

This dynamic is shaped by the joint activity of the Liver/Gall Bladder and Master of the Heart/Triple Warmer pairs. These meridians guarantee the harmonious interaction of the two poles regulating the body: the metabolic and neural centers. Their complementary activity puts the impulsive energy of the more metabolic meridians to work for the neural maturation of the individual (fig. 2.19).

MERIDIANS AND GENDER EXPRESSION

Unlike animals, human beings can achieve awareness of their sexual identity, their masculine or feminine gender. Their free will also allows them to adopt or reject this genetic reality, which is naturally modulated by the Kidneys/Bladder pair and manifests in its particular physical dimension through the Stomach/Spleen-Pancreas pair. During adolescence, the Lungs/Colon family of meridian lines becomes more active, permitting the individual to express another dimension of self—his or her virility or femininity.

The transitional period of puberty, guided by the interaction of particular secondary meridian lines—12 (Hypothalamus) and 29/09 (Gonads, that is, Ovaries or Testes)—gradually induces changes in the upper half of the body and awakens two additional secondary meridian lines, which are different for the two sexes—24 (Breasts) for women and 14 (Adam's Apple) for men.

Human beings are granted the freedom to choose their sexual expression, setting aside their biological gender. However, a number of psychophysical issues may be linked to these choices, which can or may be induced by a disrupted hormonal dynamic. In fact, the stress that accompanies the changes of puberty is presumed to disrupt the harmonious circulation of the Lungs/Colon meridians and their secondary meridian lines, which orchestrate the hormonal symphony. This can lead, for example, to a terrain that is favorable for acne, menstrual cycle problems, or food disorders, providing physical indicators of a conflicted relationship with one's gender.

While adopting one's gender is a personal process, it is also influenced by environment. Long years go into the preparation for puberty and the experience of the parental relationship has an indisputable impact on the adolescent, his or her learning process, and his or her expression of sexual identity. This is why this transition, a major step in cognitive maturation and identity building, can sometimes be difficult and create conditions that are favorable for many psychophysical disorders. It is therefore a sound move to strengthen the balance of an adolescent's vital currents that are more active during this transitional period and whose circulation is often affected by profound stress.

One specific Associative Nutripuncture method is always valuable for reinforcing the dynamics of the vital currents that are most active during puberty. Combined with the General Cellular Nutritional Regulator, it targets meridians 12 and 29/09 (female/male), as well as meridian line 24 for girls or 14 for boys, to help them accept their quickly changing bodies and discover their feminine or masculine sexual potential.

Quite often we do not take into account the immense influence of sexual expression on behavioral dynamics and the psychophysical balance of a person. The loss of identity reference points, both psychological and sexual, experienced by many people has demonstrated the influence that the hormonal dynamic, which is often disrupted, has on the expression of sexual identity. However, a person can reveal their male or female potential at any age. For expressing their personality in accord with their sexual potential, women can use an Associative Nutripuncture that stimulates meridian lines 24 (Breasts) and 07 (Vagina). Men can stimulate meridians 14 (Adam's Apple) and 06 (Penis); both genders should combine these individualized treatments with the General Cellular Nutritional Regulator.

Even during and after menopause, women can stimulate these same meridians to adjust the irritations that accompany the hormonal changes taking place, which can subject their emotional equilibrium to a severe ordeal. In part 3 of the book, you will find more details on the action of Sequential Nutripuncture during these crucial stages of life.

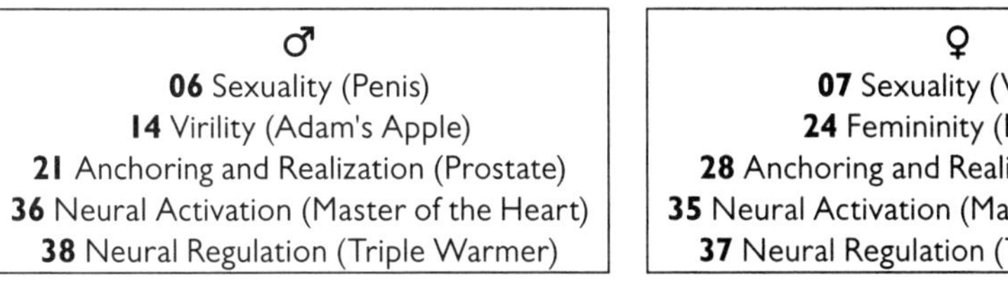

♂	♀
06 Sexuality (Penis)	**07** Sexuality (Vagina)
14 Virility (Adam's Apple)	**24** Femininity (Breasts)
21 Anchoring and Realization (Prostate)	**28** Anchoring and Realization (Uterus)
36 Neural Activation (Master of the Heart)	**35** Neural Activation (Master of the Heart)
38 Neural Regulation (Triple Warmer)	**37** Neural Regulation (Triple Warmer)

Fig. 2.20. Five Sexual Meridians

3
Four Vital Parameters for the Body, Four Essential Conditions for Ensuring Its Vitality

EXPERIMENTS PERFORMED over many years have made it possible to discover the fundamental parameters governing the balance of all life-forms, knowledge that the present has forgotten despite how essential it is to our well-being. This knowledge consists of four simple yet complex references that provide essential landmarks for the coherent expression of every individual. These are internal reference points that allow us to interact in an optimum way with our environment while still respecting our particular sensibilities.

Four Vital Parameters of the Body

1. Bipolarity (positive yin-yang), which guarantees the vitality of cellular exchanges
2. Fitting into a given space and time; being in the here and now
3. Spatial orientation, coordinating our gestures and guiding effective action
4. Sensory and cognitive identity, which positions us in relation to those around us and refines our ability to communicate with ourselves and with others

---

Going from the simplest to the most complex, we are going to take a look at just what these parameters are and the role they play in our everyday dynamics.

1. ***Bipolarity (positive yin-yang), which guarantees the vitality of cellular exchanges.*** First, it should be pointed out that life (on the organic or mental cellular level) is always the result of the interaction of two opposing poles, which are complementary at the same time, that animate our minds and bodies: yin (metabolic, feminine force) and yang (cerebral masculine force). The principle of yin and yang—the recognition of two interdependent energies and their interactions and relationship—is of core importance in Eastern traditions. It is obviously a metaphor for identifying the complementary/opposing activity of the systems ensuring our vitality: nerve center/blood center, arterial/vein circulation, right brain/left brain, cerebral center/sexual center, and so forth. Each of these two inseparable poles is essential for the other's expression; their synergy is the prime support of life. When the activity of these two poles is not synchronous—in other words, when one system gains the upper hand over the other—it produces a sense that something is not right physically or mentally, which can lead to deep metabolic or neural disorders. This means that the most basic balance to monitor is the *bipolar dynamic,* what in Nutripuncture we call "positive yin-yang."

   When this fundamental parameter is in place, every pole interacts coherently with its complementary pole, acknowledging and mutually cooperating with each other to ensure the harmonious circulation of the vital currents. The result? Optimum vitality. An acupuncturist might tell you that you are thus in the Tao; you are meshed with a context, field, or milieu that is favorable to life and allows it to develop, evolve, and manifest its potential. Once this parameter's stability is assured, which is of major importance for our cells, life needs to become anchored in a specific space during a specific time.
2. ***Fitting into a given space and time; being in the here and now.*** Being able to fit into our space-time allows us to be present in the moment. This parameter is as important as the first. In addition to a coherent bipolar dynamic, our cells also require the correct calibration of factors relating to pressure and temperature. Pressure defines the gravitational field our cells occupy and in which our activities occur; it gives them the weight they need to anchor themselves in

place. This extends to larger structures as well, such as the uterus, the prostate, the knees, and the skeletal structure, which are very sensitive to gravitational information. These structures are often stressed, congested, and weakened when moving out of a home or traveling. It has also been observed that the thyroid is quite sensitive to jet lag and that during an intercontinental trip, for example, its meridian line 27 is often disrupted by the irritations caused by time changes.

The notion of time (defined by light intensity and temperature) is essential for our cells, because it scans the rhythmic information necessary to orchestrate the sequence of biological functions such as the cyclical production of hormones.

3. ***Spatial orientation, coordinating our gestures and guiding effective action.*** The notion of spatial orientation allows us to easily get our bearings in the surrounding space. This is the third parameter that plays an important role in the quality of our lives. Being able to identify right and left without difficulty is, for example, a sign of balance and coordination. In fact, when we are well oriented, our gestures are efficient and do not incur much cost to our energy levels. However, our individual corporeal diagram (the blueprint of the body the brain uses to command our gestures) does not always conform to anatomical reality and sometimes the architectural depiction of our body is crammed with logistical errors. We confuse high and low, right and left, the hip with the knee, the ankle with the wrist, and so on; confusing their functions produces short circuits that can affect our performance. The coordination of our gestures actually depends on the motor patterns we constructed during earliest childhood, such as learning to walk, which does not always take place in the best possible emotional and sensory conditions. This can create various mental and physical problems, hence the importance of dynamizing the meridians involved in the essential faculty of spatial orientation. This allows us to "update" our body diagram to conform to anatomical reality.
4. ***Sensory and cognitive identity, which positions us in relation to those around us and refines our ability to communicate with ourselves and with others.*** In other words being oneself, and feeling comfortable as a man or woman in all circumstances, is also an essential parameter for ensuring a harmonious psychophysical dynamic. The notion of identity is physically obvious if we stop and consider

that we all have distinctive physiognomies and a unique fingerprint. However, identity also expresses itself through the sensory perception unique to every individual, which permits us to evaluate life in accordance with our own sensibilities. Identity can be defined as the central axis of an individual's mental and gestural expression. It is an ongoing process, an open and dynamic system that is constantly changing under the stimulus of experience. It is the aptitude of maintaining an identity while still evolving and changing from contact with the environment.

In fact each of us needs to differentiate ourselves to better know ourselves, build ourselves, assert ourselves, enrich ourselves, love, and exist. Difference is the basis of the desire dwelling within all people: the desire for exchange and communication, for sharing and discovering what is different from oneself. Cultivating the benchmarks of our identity is in large part what ensures our mental and physical vitality.

THE NOTION OF BIPOLARITY: THE YIN-YANG BALANCE

According to Eastern traditions, life is governed by the permanent interaction between the two inseparable forces of yin and yang, which can be pictured as scales that regulate the dynamic organization of the living being. The yin-yang dynamic is a basic, essential condition to guarantee our overall vitality; it ensures the viability of our sensory perception and makes us become more aware of our natural and human environment, while building better physical and mental health.

Yin is a more metabolic and feminine force related to blood while yang is a more cerebral masculine force related to the nerves. Bipolarity is an evolutionary constant that can be found in all biological expression: acid-alkaline, nerve center-blood center, sympathetic and parasympathetic nervous system, male-female, and so on. The meridians also function as couples, as we will later see in detail. The interaction of two opposing poles is indispensable for the birth, maturation, and maintaining of life. It can be seen everywhere, at every level.

Cellular Yin-Yang

On the cellular level this yin-yang bipolarity is exhibited by differences in membrane potential, which activate exchanges and communications between all cells.

The Cellular Membrane Under the Microscope

The cytoplasmic membrane is organized in a double layer made up of lipids and protides. It resembles a fluid mosaic, formed from proteins floating like icebergs on an ocean of lipids. The lipid composition of the inner and outer single layers is not identical. This reflects the functional difference of the two surfaces of the cellular membrane.

The external layer is the cell's communication surface between the extra cellular fluid and the interface of the other cells. It holds special properties that sets it apart and allows it to communicate with the outside world. Specific molecules facilitate this communication: glycolipids and glycoproteins. These two are genuine markers of cellular identity because they are derived from galactose.

The glycolipids ensure cellular adhesion as well as the recognition and the communication among cells. The glycoproteins support the selective entrance of certain substances. This dynamic induces an electric potential difference at the membrane level, necessary for ionic exchanges and balanced cellular nutrition.

Bruce Lipton, a biologist at Stanford University, has shown through his research the importance of these membrane level exchanges for cellular vitality and self-regulation, which he believes to be as fundamental as the central action of DNA.

Every change occurring in the environment is likely to modify the membrane

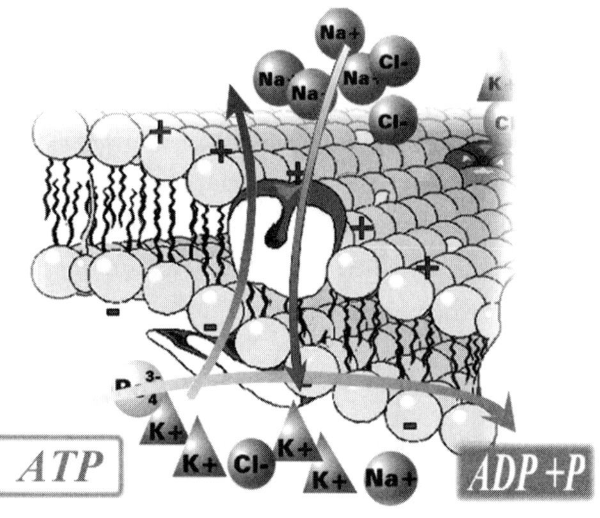

Fig. 3.1. Nutri Yin–Nutri Yang encourages cellular communication and supports overall bipolar (yin-yang) balance.

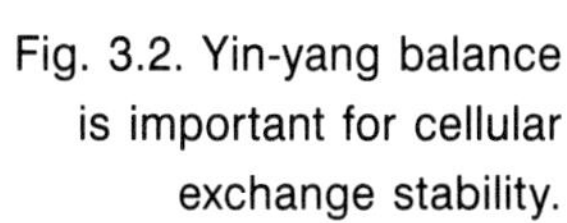

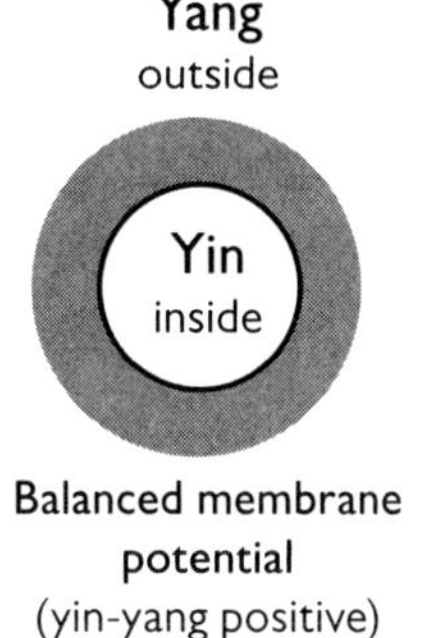

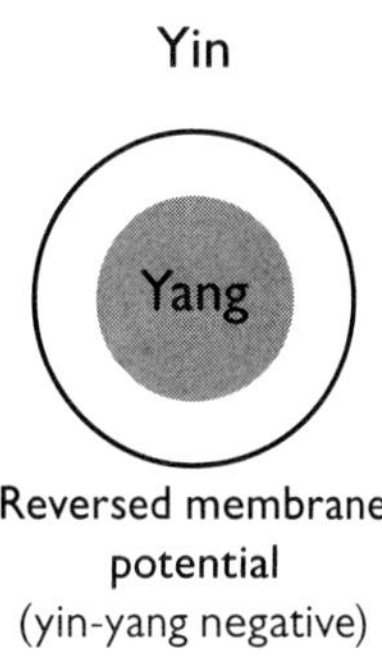

Fig. 3.2. Yin-yang balance is important for cellular exchange stability.

potential. The difference in potential between the inner layer and the outer layer of cellular membranes creates an "inside-outside" orientation and a polarization that plays a determining role in the entire organism's vital processes. In situations of physical or mental fatigue, exchanges are disturbed and the membrane potentials are decreased, even reversed (fig. 3.2); hence the importance of reinforcing it as a form of prevention for cellular exchange stability. It is therefore wise to support the bipolar (yin-yang) balance of these two layers and restore sufficient membrane potential to ensure the dynamics of these exchanges.

In Nutripuncture, we use the General Cellular Nutritional Regulator, a fundamental nutritional supplement, to activate all cellular communication in an optimal

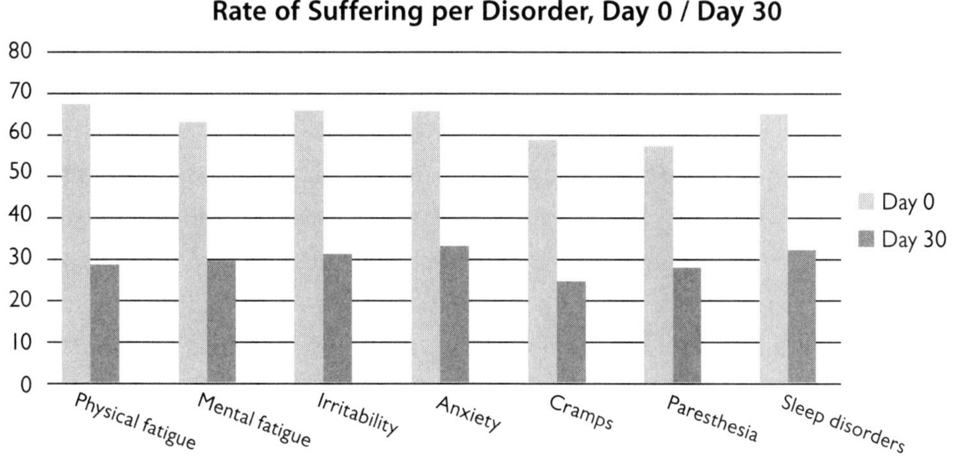

Fig. 3.3. Research on the effects of the General Cellular Nutritional Regulator on sleep quality, excitability, and physical and mental fatigue

way, thus restoring the tone and calm required to maintain optimal vitality. It can be taken at any age and has proven to be particularly effective in correcting deficiencies for weakened people, school-age children and toddlers, pregnant women, those who experience extremely stressful lives, the elderly, students, athletes . . . pretty much everyone you can think of. During a period of convalescence, it allows for a faster recovery. It is particularly helpful during times of physical or psychological stress, at the onset of a disease, convalescence, or in the event of a decline in form, morale, or tonicity.

Research on the General Cellular Nutritional Regulator

A study is currently under way on the isolated hippocampus cells of rats. To begin, injection of a picrotoxin, which made them "epileptics" harmed these cells. The layout of the membrane potential showed great synchronous and rhythmic electric shocks. The second time, we added the GCNR and after a few minutes observed an improvement of the condition, with significant reduction in the amplitude and frequency of the discharges.

Yin-Yang Balance of Metabolic and Nerve Activity

In the first chapter we mentioned that the meridian network has key points that allow the many circuits to communicate, like the stations of a subway system of a major city. Among the key points in the body there are two large regulation centers. Like traffic cops, they control the flow of the information from the meridian lines from the lower half of the body, which are more metabolic in nature, into the meridians of the upper half, which are more neural.

These two centers, strategic opposites and essential complements, are crossroads toward which travel all the information that describes the state—balanced or not—of the other organs. Their role is to sponge up excesses, regulate deficits, and encourage the overall harmony of the vital current network. Providing us with food and wisdom, their harmonious synergy triggers a dual process, resulting in a stable vital force and a calm mental attitude. These inseparable poles form a site of profound exchange, where the biological and the mental meet, dialogue, cooperate, and mutually influence each other.

The yang cerebral pole is formed of meridian line 08 of Cerebral Cortex and meridian lines 35/36 of the Master of the Heart and 37/38 of the Triple Warmer;

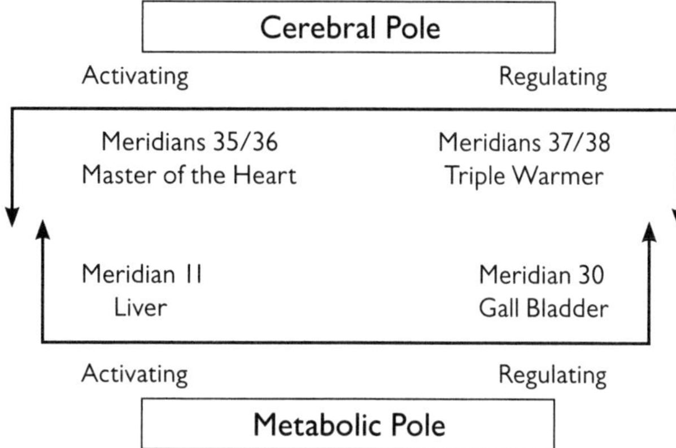

Fig. 3.4. The yang cerebral pole and the yin metabolic pole regulate the flow of information from the lower half of the body to the upper half.

the yin metabolic pole is formed of Liver meridian line 11 and Gall Bladder meridian line 30. When all the organs, nourished by balanced yin-yang, are functioning as a coherent unit, the Cerebral Cortex will be better able to perform its job as pilot, analyzing and directing the dynamics of the entire body. The Liver, the preeminent metabolic center, provides the necessary fuel to guarantee vitality of the organism, thanks to its production of A.T.P. and its glycogen reserves.

Every time the organism is subjected to a stress or a demanding task, certain meridian lines are weakened, which affect these two poles. This is how a disturbance of the Stomach or Pancreas can disturb the Liver or the cerebral pole. By stimulating the dynamics of the meridian lines that control these two poles, we support their capacity for self-regulation and improving general psychophysical balance.

The Yang Cerebral Pole: Meridian Line 08 of Cognitive Integration, Meridian Lines 35/36 of the Master of the Heart and 37/38 of the Triple Warmer

One of the principal functions of the Cerebral Cortex is the memory setting of the information accumulated by the life experience of the cells of each organic system. This function can be disturbed by the quality and the quantity of the information received by its meridian lines, but also by the dysfunction of other meridian lines. Meridian line 08 partners with the meridian lines 35/36 and 37/38 that rule the sympathetic and parasympathetic nervous systems. The interaction of these meridian lines is paramount to ensure the body's neural conduction as well as the balance of our minds.

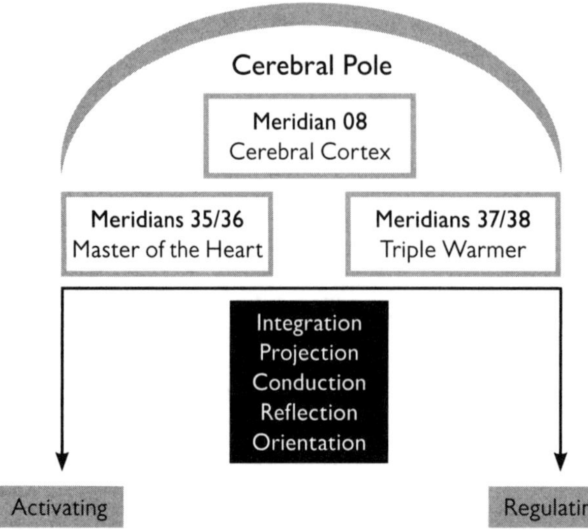

Fig. 3.5. The interaction of meridian lines 08, 35/36, and 37/38 is paramount to ensure the balance of our minds.

The Yin Metabolic Pole: Meridian Lines Liver 11 and Gall Bladder 30

We know that the Liver is the energy reservoir of the organism; it is a true energy center. Disruption of its meridians can entail a decline of vitality and engender a state of fatigue, or sometimes aggressive behavior. Meridian line 11 acts as a metabolic regulator. Its stimulation is recommended in the event of general exhaustion, often combined with meridian line 08.

The Gallbladder plays a fundamental role in the emulsion of fats. Meridian line 30, the partner of meridian line 11, is often to blame in liver and lipidic disorders. Its regulation can offer a sense of well-being to anxious and worried people.

To sum up: the body is not a group of isolated systems but the result of the synergy of various functions, which can acknowledge each other (balanced yin-yang dynamic) or ignore each other (reversed yang-yin dynamic). Each meridian line

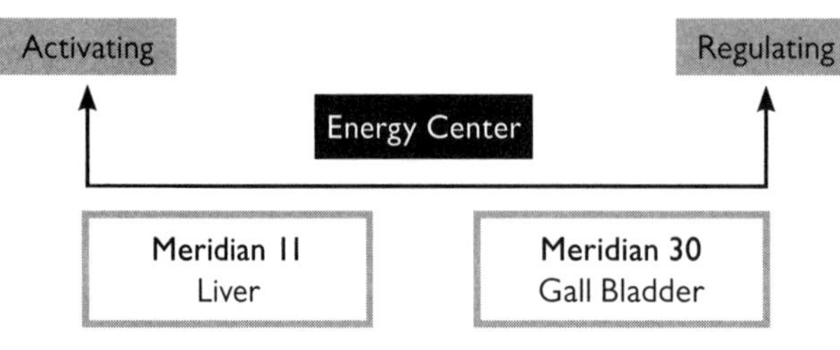

Fig. 3.6. Partner meridians 11 and 30 are key to vitality and well-being.

is interactive: it communicates its information to other meridians and forms part of a complex network in which all the impulses necessary for the body's self-regulation circulate. For example, an emotional shock can disrupt information that governs the balance of the Heart meridian line to the point of generating a depressive state or irritable behavior, betraying the interference of meridian line 04 (Heart) with meridian line 11. Jointly nourishing the more weakened meridians makes it possible to overcome severe stress, which left alone can make the cellular terrain more favorable for deeper disorders.

When each meridian combines and interacts consistently with the others, vital equilibrium is ensured. However, the complexity of the body is such that this balance is always unstable due to the fact that each of us is an open system in a permanent dynamic with our environment. Supporting our vitality is therefore essential.

FITTING INTO A TIME AND PLACE: A MATTER OF RHYTHM AND LIGHT

While we have not quite determined what information modulates cellular rhythm, it is obvious that the notion of time is connected with our perception. A child perceives time differently from an old person and the rhythm that punctuates the cellular life of an embryo is completely different from that of an adult organism. There probably is a relationship with cellular metabolism, given rhythm by the biological clocks that are so plentiful in our bodies. The synchronized activity of our various biological clocks is given rhythm by luminous information (the intensity of the exposure to light and the times at which that exposure takes place).

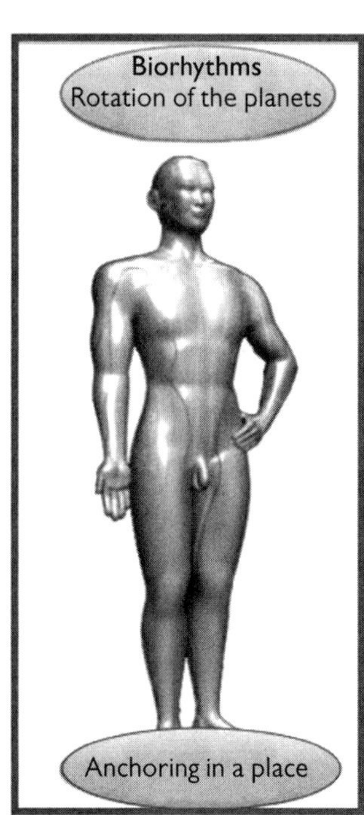

Fig. 3.7. Fitting into a time and place

These clocks, called "oscillators," are numerous and provide the rhythm for the cycle of the different body functions. Just as in the works of a clock, in which there are wheels that revolve at different speeds, the functions in the body have their own rhythms, although all are keyed to a single biological time. Studies of chronobiology have made it possible to understand an entire series of physiological anomalies caused by the poor coordination of biorhythms as well as the difficulties they cause in physical and intellectual adaptation, which prevent us from being in the "here and now."

Chronobiology has listed different rhythms such as circadian rhythm and ultradian rhythms. A circadian rhythm is an endogenously driven twenty-four-hour cycle of some of our biological functions, of which the waking/sleeping cycle is the most important. Under normal conditions, this alternation is synchronized by the rhythm of day/night, and our resting/working activities.

With respect to circadian rhythms, there are two principle oscillators (fig. 3.8):

A strong oscillator, which is stable and barely affected by environmental changes. Its nature is primarily metabolic. It adjusts body temperature, the REM sleep stage, and the release of certain hormones (such as cortisol). It is regarded in Nutripuncture as yin.

A weak oscillator, which functions rapidly and is much more sensitive to time and to signals coming from the environment. It synchronizes our sleep and waking rhythms and probably governs some nocturnal secretions like melatonin, prolactin, and growth hormone. It can readily go out of order but it also makes it possible to adapt fairly quickly to time changes. According to Nutripuncture research, this oscillator is regarded as yang.

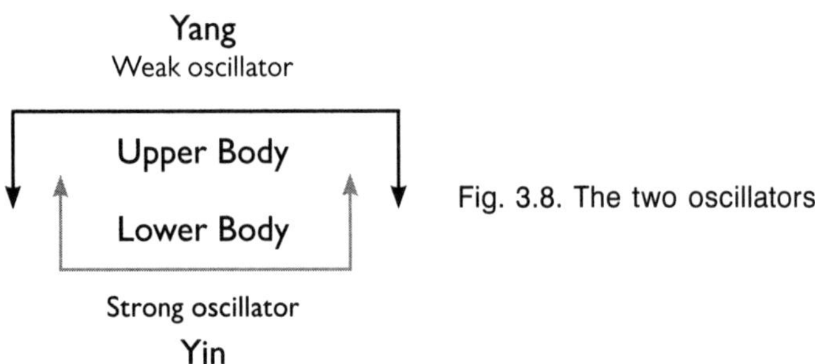

Fig. 3.8. The two oscillators

Many forms of stress—such as long flights, night or long work shifts, and also, quite simply, drastic seasonal changes—can throw these oscillators out of order, which can disrupt the harmonious sequence of cellular functions, manifested by difficulties in fitting in and feeling anchored in a place (fig. 3.9). Individual sensitivity to these external rhythmic modifications varies. Some need a few days to adapt, others sometimes weeks. It has been observed that this adaptation becomes more challenging after thirty-five years of age, especially in depressive subjects or those who have psychological problems. It is also difficult for young children.

In response to such changes, the weak oscillator—which has an impact on the waking/sleep cycle—quickly tunes in with the environment. We are able to quickly (in two or three days) adjust our alertness, waking up and falling asleep according to the solar rhythm of a new location, for example. On the other hand, the strong oscillator—which is related to cortisol release and body temperature—is less responsive to the environment and requires a much longer time to adjust to a new living condition. For several days, maybe even several weeks, internal synchronization will not be established, causing fatigue, dizziness, and difficulty in sleeping.

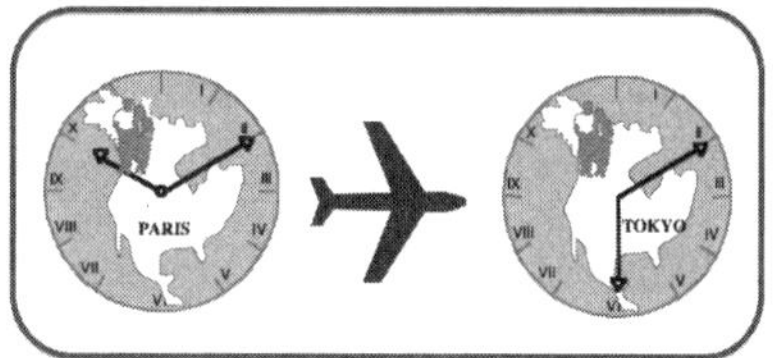

Fig. 3.9. Stressors such as time change can disrupt cellular functions.

The ultradian rhythms—recurrent periods or cycles repeated throughout a twenty-four-hour circadian day—represent shorter periods from only a few minutes to a couple of hours, also shaping our days and nights. Thus, during sleep, periods of dreaming and dreamless sleep follow one another. In the course of the day, we observe alternated cycles of activity and rest, great effectiveness and tiredness, phases of active wakefulness during which we are very alert, and phases of passive wakefulness during which we are less sharp, less effective. These rhythms influence the majority of our biological functions such as cardiac and respiration, our internal body temperature and our hormonal secretions. They influence our physical and mental performances; we are very familiar with the feelings of fatigue we experience around lunchtime, from 1 to 2 p.m., whereas most of us generally feel in top form around 5 p.m.

Our Diurnal Cycle

All that lives has a cyclical rhythm: birth, maturation, and death. Some cycles are short while others are long. There are the different sleep cycles that take place in one night, the menstrual cycle of women, the cycle of the seasons over the course of the year, the phases of the moon, and other various annual and biannual cycles.

The human being is a diurnal animal because its biological rhythms are punctuated by light and the alternation of day and night. Human performance levels are at their maximum during certain hours of the day depending on the circulation of certain meridians.

For example, the performance of the central nervous system (attention, motor coordination, memory, etc.), as well as muscle strength and cardiac and respiratory frequencies, reach their maximum levels over the course of the day.

Conversely, other biological variations, such as the rate of lymphocytes (white blood cells that play a role in the body's defenses against infection) have their maximum level of activity during the middle of the night.

Spatial-Temporal Anchoring: Being Present in the Here and Now

The notion of spatial anchoring is a fundamental parameter for ensuring our vitality. The meridians adjust for the impact of the magnetic field of the places we live and work. When they are stressed, our actions will be ineffective, insubstantial, and ungrounded. When we are not anchored, our potential for action cannot manifest and we have a hard time moving forward—in short, we are treading water. Hence the importance of supporting the circulation of the meridians that modulate our anchoring to a place—to ensure the quality and the effectiveness of our actions.

Temporal anchoring, being in the present, is also a fundamental parameter for our vitality, as it gives rhythm to activity. When we are out of step, we have trouble managing our time, we find it hard to be in the moment and present to self and others. For example, attention deficit problems, which are fairly frequent with school age children, are often connected to a poor fit in the time and place one is living.

In Nutripuncture, meridian 27, which governs the Thyroid and time, plays a fundamental role in the overall balance of organic rhythms and coordinates inner biological clocks with a given timeframe. It constitutes an essential reference for

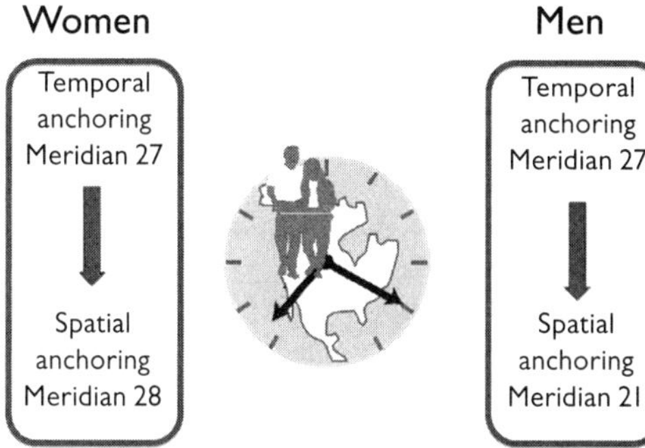

Fig. 3.10. The joint invigoration of meridians 27 and 28 (for women) or 27 and 21 (for men) is always advisable after a move, a trip, or during travel to ensure a high performance level, such as for an athlete or a singer, whose voice is the mirror of his or her vitality. It is also of value to those people whose heads "are always in the clouds" and never seem to find a good fit with the "here and now," and whose actions thereby lack effectiveness.

everyone, much as the Greenwich Meridian represents a temporal landmark for Europeans. This is why after a transatlantic flight it is just as important to adjust this meridian as it is to change the time on our watch. Doing so will make it possible for our bodies to more quickly capture and harness the information connected with the light and outside temperature, integrate them, and adapt accordingly.

All temporal adaptations presume finding a good fit with a new place so we can set roots there, even if only temporarily. It is therefore recommended to conjointly activate the meridians of anchoring and material action: meridian 28 of the Uterus for women or 21 of the Prostate for men. It is also recommended to start being active right away (jogging, walking, eating) in accordance with the new time, and eat meals consisting of the local specialties.

The Rhythms of the Meridians: Nychthemeral (Daily) Rhythms

According to the Eastern tradition, each family of meridian lines is more active at certain hours of the day and during certain seasons.

In acupuncture, the practitioner is very knowledgeable about the variation of meridian activity according to the time of day (fig. 3.11; see also color insert). This dynamic concept is also found in the description of nychthemeral rhythm where, every two hours, a meridian line is particularly activated. For example, at 3:00 a.m. the "energy tide" reaches the meridian line of the Lung (meridian line 20); ironically, this is the traditional time for asthma attacks to occur.

Each meridian plays a part in the general circulation of the body's vital currents. When the circulation of a meridian line is disturbed, it will no longer be in tune with the others. It is thus necessary to regulate it so that it is properly synchronized with the rhythms of the body so it can recover its proper place, role, and all its vitality. Using Nutripuncture you can recover this synchronization quickly and restore the vital currents.

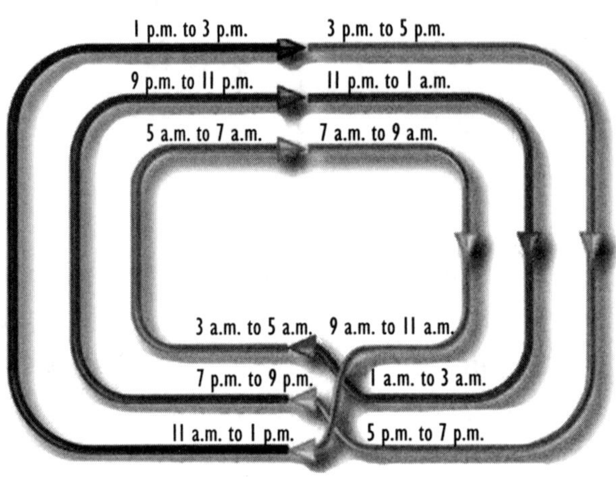

3:00 a.m. to 5:00 a.m. Lung meridian line 20 (Shou Tai Yin)
5:00 a.m. to 7:00 a.m. Colon meridian line 05 (Shou Yang Ming)
7:00 a.m. to 9:00 a.m. Stomach meridian line 10 (Zu Yang Ming)
9:00 a.m. to 11:00 a.m. Spleen-Pancreas meridian line 18 (Zu Tai Yin)
11:00 a.m. to 1:00 p.m. Heart meridian line 04 (Shou Shao Yin)
1:00 p.m. to 3:00 p.m. Small Intestine meridian line 13 (Shou Tai Yang)
3:00 p.m. to 5:00 p.m. Bladder meridian line 31 (Zu Tai Yang)
5:00 p.m. to 7:00 p.m. Kidney meridian line 22 (Zu Shao Yin)
7:00 p.m. to 9:00 p.m. Master of the Heart meridian lines 35/36 (Shou Jue Yin)
9:00 p.m. to 11:00 p.m. Triple Warmer meridian lines 37/38 (Shou Shao Yang)
11:00 p.m. to 1:00 a.m. Gall Bladder meridian line 30 (Zu Shao Yang)
1:00 a.m. to 3:00 a.m. Liver meridian line 11 (Zu Jue Yin)

Fig. 3.11. Circadian rhythm of the meridians

Seasonal Rhythms, Organic Rhythms

The rotation of the earth around the sun determines the seasons. According to the Eastern tradition, each season activates a family of meridian lines whose activity flourishes at a certain time of the year and heightens the sensitivity of the senses they nourish (fig. 3.12). If this choreography is not synchronous with nature's rhythms,

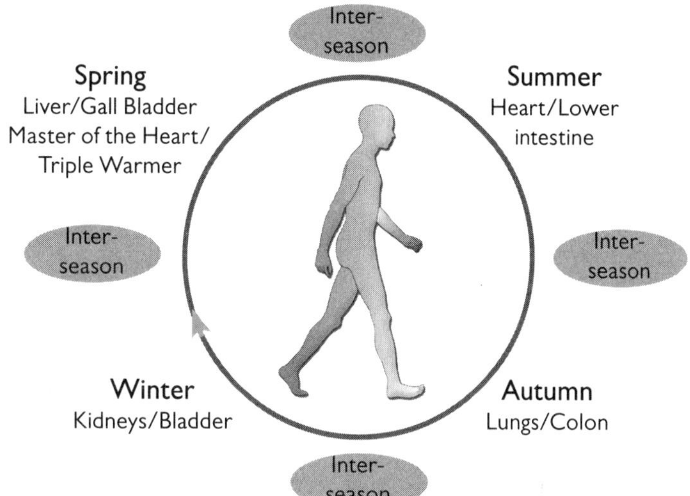

Fig. 3.12. Each season activates a family of meridian lines whose activity flourishes at a certain time of the year.

circadian flows, seasonal cycles, or certain biological functions (hormonal secretions, alternation between being awake/asleep), our psychophysical balance can be weakened.

The Meridian Lines of Summer: The Heart/Small Intestine Family

According to Eastern tradition, our vitality at this time of year depends on the ability of the vital currents of the Heart/Small Intestine family to regulate their activities. In synergy with other secondary meridian lines, they govern the sense of sight.

- Meridian line 04 of the Heart supports the rhythm system of the communication ensured by meridian line 01 of the Arteries (complementary to meridian line 29 of the Veins in the Kidneys/Bladder family). They also help maintain emotional balance.
- Meridian line 13 of the Small Intestine regulates the quality of assimilation. If immune disorders are present, it is vital to regulate them.
- Meridian line 01 of the Arteries governs the circulatory impulse ensured by the heart.
- Meridian line 32 of Vision provides support to the faculty of looking.
- Meridian line 08 of the Cerebral Cortex ensures the balance of the sensitive neural pole in its role as the body's orchestra conductor. It adjusts the individual's mental projections, shaped by his or her outlook.

Between Seasons

In addition to the four seasons, the Eastern tradition places between each season a transitional period, called *inter-season* or *seasonal cusp*, which marks the passage from one season to another (the first and last week of every season). At the end of the summer (from about August 15 to September 20), this transition phase is more intense and constitutes a season of its own: late summer.

The Meridians of the End of Summer: The Stomach/Spleen-Pancreas Family

The seasonal transition that takes place at the end of summer is characterized by the growing potency of the vital currents of the Stomach/Spleen-Pancreas family, the master meridian lines of this period and to which other secondary meridian lines are attached.

- Meridian line 18 of the Pancreas oversees optimal transformation of food and the incorporation of the energy needed for cellular function.
- Meridian line 28 of the Uterus makes it possible to express the will to live, to transform one's plans into reality, and to generate a job or a baby.
- Meridian line 21 of the Prostate also makes it possible to express the desire to live, work, and engender life.
- Meridian 26 of the Thalamus (in connection with the central gray matter) regulates the cerebral core that directs and controls action, and movement in general.
- Meridian 17 of Bone adjusts the density of the skeletal structure. The expression: "to have nerve" characterizes this vital current.
- Meridian line 16 of the Muscles ensures the dynamic of the muscle and bone system. Although this meridian line is part of the Lungs/Colon family, its circulation can be invigorated this time of year because they share with the meridian line of Bone the job of overseeing structural and postural balance.

The Meridian Lines of Autumn: The Lungs/Colon Family

The passage of autumn is characterized by the activation of the vital currents of the Lungs/Colon pair, master meridian lines for this season to which are attached a number of secondary meridians.

- Meridian line 20 of the Lungs ensures balanced exchanges with the ambient air, expressing confidence, and ensuring mental flexibility.
- Meridian line 05 of the Colon expresses the ability to organize, and regulates elimination of metabolic wastes.
- Meridian line 25 of the Sinus and meridian line 12 of the Hypothalamus regulate the sense of smell.
- Meridian line 15 of the Lymphatic system oversees the dynamic of the immune system.
- Meridian line 14 of the Adam's Apple (in men) begins activating the expression of virility from the time of puberty.
- Meridian line 24 of the Breasts (for women) regulates the expression of femininity.
- Meridian lines 07 of the Vagina (for women) and 06 of the Penis (for men) controls the dynamic of sex life.
- Meridian line 16 of the Muscles encourages the flexibility and elasticity necessary for movement.

The Meridian Lines of Winter: The Kidneys/Bladder Family

The duration of winter is characterized by the activation of the vital currents of the Kidneys/Bladder couple, to which are connected several other secondary meridian lines.

- Meridian line 22 of the Kidneys governs the balance of fluid exchanges. If we are to consider the Kidney meridian line as the guarantor of assurance, the meridian line of the Bladder is attributed with an influence over alertness.
- Meridian line 31 of the Bladder is one of the most complex circuits of the body. Acupuncture assigns a very important role to this meridian line, which is quite different from the role played by the organ to which it is attached, which Western science considers a simple reservoir. This meridian line, located on a line almost in the middle of the back, includes points that reflect the condition of every sector of the body.
- Meridian line 29 of the Veins regulates the balance of the blood returning from the arteries. This is the meridian of receptivity.
- Meridian line 02 of the Cerebellum governs muscle tone and postural balance.

- Meridian line 09 of the Adrenal Glands ensures the circulation of ancestral energy. This is a meridian of the "source."
- Meridian line 23 of the Retina permits reception of the image in accordance with the projected gaze. It is the meridian of representation.
- Meridian line 27 of the Thyroid governs temporal anchoring.
- The joint action of meridian lines 09 and 29, the Gonads, ensures the continuity of the species.

The Meridian Lines of Spring: The Liver/Gall Bladder Family and the Master of the Heart/Triple Warmer Family

Spring is when nature reawakens with the rise of new sap in all the plants. Human beings share a similar rise in the potency of the metabolic (blood) pole, which is normally contained and limited by the cerebral (neural) pole. The meridian lines 11 (Liver) and 30 (Gall Bladder) regulate the metabolic blood impulse. In synergy with the Master of the Heart and Triple Warmer meridians, they govern the sense of touch.

The meridian lines of the Master of the Heart and the Triple Warmer polarize the cognitive expression of the individual in accordance with his or her gender. This is why in Nutripuncture there are female Master of the Heart meridian lines (35) or male lines (36), and female Triple Warmer meridian lines (37) and male ones (38).

The meridian lines 19 (Skin) and 03 (Hair), which ensure tactile equilibrium and the integrity of skin appendages in general, are secondary meridian lines of this double family.

FINDING YOUR BEARINGS WITHOUT LOSING YOUR HEAD

Right or left? Do you have trouble getting oriented? Do you have good stable landmarks in your personal space? Can you master laterality without having to stop and think? How many times have you gone astray when driving or giving directions to lost tourists? And again why do you sometimes feel so clumsy, disoriented, and out of it?

To get our bearings in the space around us, our bodies rely on proprioception (the ability to perceive ourselves internally), which is entirely a reflex action and one we develop very early in life, from the time we make our first movements as a baby. As we learn to walk, depending on the stimuli the brain receives from the movement, we build in our heads a kind of topographical map that locates all the sectors of the body and provides a diagram for guiding our gestures (fig. 3.13). This virtual diagram takes place in the brain three dimensionally (up-down, right-left, front-back) and reproduces each sector of the body in accordance with its anatomical position, an essential and strategic step for guaranteeing its function.

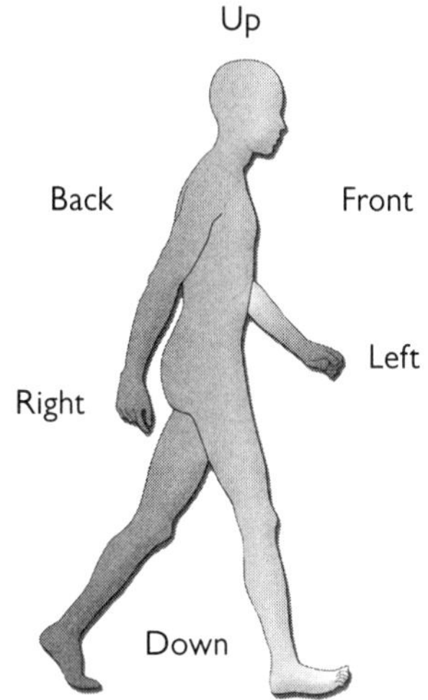

Fig. 3.13. Spatial orientation

This is how our cognitive abilities develop individually, based on the awareness we acquire of our body's architecture, the perception of its movements (proprioception), and by virtue of the information we receive through our five senses. However many people, even adults, display problems with lateralization and spatial disorientation, connected with a poorly drawn body diagram from early childhood or one thrown into disorder by serious stress (accident, shock). With the help of different tests, we have observed that the localization of a joint or appendage in the body diagram does not always correspond with its actual anatomical position. This provides favorable conditions for a loss of motor coordination, exhaustion, or various disorders that are sometimes difficult to identify.

I remember a person suffering from a problem in his right knee that began after a long hike in the mountains. He had been given a number of different tests but the cause had not been discovered. We naturally suggested he stimulate the meridians connected with the knee: no result. When we saw him again several days later, he told us that his hip was beginning to give him trouble. With the help of a test on his body diagram, we found that he was actually confusing his knee and his hip. We also noticed an erroneous walking dynamic whose motor was the knee instead of the pelvis. Once his hip meridians had been stimulated for several weeks, his knee felt much better and his hips had relearned their job as motor function. The way he walked became more fluid and easy.

When someone has misused a joint, to the point its function has deviated off course, the circulation of the corresponding vital currents will also have been detoured, over time inducing functional troubles, then lesions, sometimes with no apparent cause. Indeed, the various corporeal benchmarks (among which the joints play a major role) form an essential base for providing effectiveness, strength, and coordination to our gestures and for building a harmonious relationship to the space around us.

Everyone knows the importance of lateralization, the ability to tell right from left, for which there is no lack of practical examples. On the other hand, when we consider the mental representation of the dimensions of front and back, we come across metaphors like "moving forward," as opposed to "taking a step backward," or even "projecting oneself into the future" or "stuck in the past." Learning to differentiate these opposing-complementary dimensions makes it possible, for example, to improve our way of walking and advancing through life. This is why, when we project our bodies forward in accord with a mental projection going in the same direction, we increase the coordination of our steps and move forward more effectively, quickly, and pleasantly. Metaphorically, this allows us to project ourselves into life differently, especially when we think we are getting ahead but are unconsciously doing everything in our power to go backward. Up and down, synonyms for climbing and descending, similarly form fundamental spatial landmarks for the mind as well as the body.

Our representation of our self, our body image, is therefore a fundamental

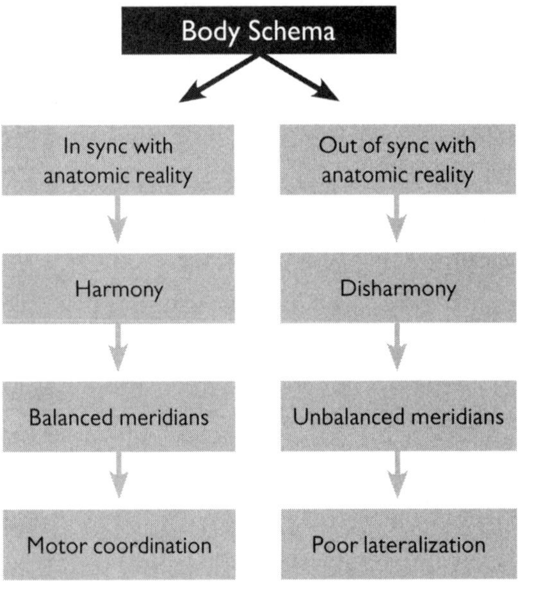

Fig. 3.14. Our motor coordination (or lack thereof) is a result of our awareness (or lack thereof) of our body's architecture.

parameter that ensures a healthy and authentic relationship between the mind and body, which is essential for our physical and mental vitality. The vital currents involved in the faculty of spatial orientation are two "highways" that emerge from the level of the perineum and ascend to the head (they end at the mouth). The course of the Conception Vessel, meridian line 33, outlines the median front line of the body, and that of the Governor Vessel, meridian line 34, outlines the back median line (fig. 3.15). The Conception/Governor couple therefore connects the top and bottom of the body, its right and left, and its front and back, thereby defining its three spatial dimensions.

Another pair of meridian lines, partner to this Conception/Governor couple, define a fourth dimension—inside and outside—which is essential for our spatial organization (fig. 3.16). These are the Master of the Heart (35 for women, 36 for men) and Triple Warmer (37 for women, 38 for men), which play an important role in differentiating the inner space of the body and its outer surface, essential in the depiction of our body!

Jointly supporting the circulation of these four "sentinel" meridian lines, in addition to thereby ensuring overall psychophysical balance, is recommended in

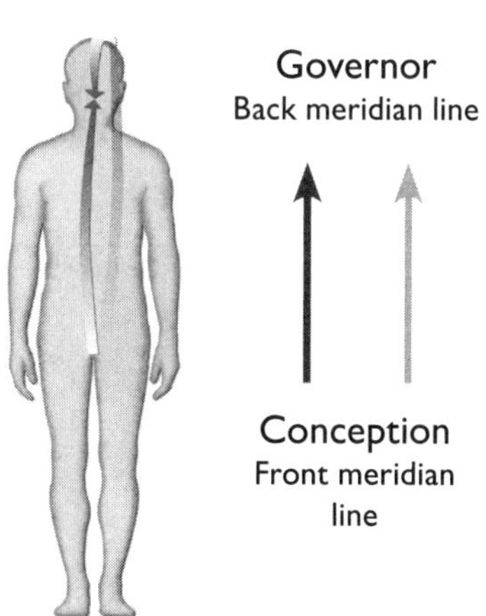

Fig. 3.15. The Conception and Governor lines define the body's three spatial dimensions.

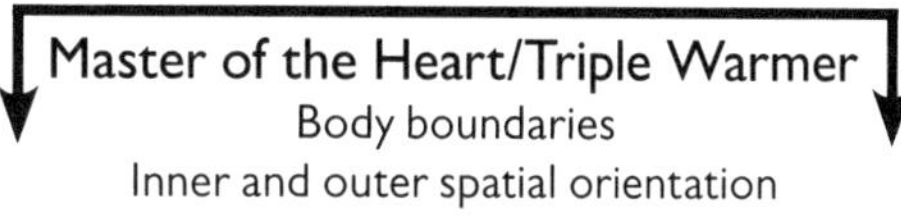

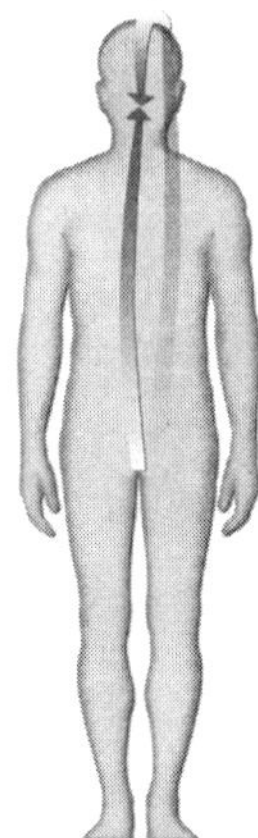

Fig. 3.16. The Master of the Heart and Triple Warmer meridian lines play an important role in differentiating the inner space of the body from its outer surface.

the case of stress and chronic fatigue, which can make us feel as if we are upside down, disoriented, and out of it, which causes a sudden sharp drop in our vitality. Meridian lines 33 Conception and 34 Governor, like actual highways, make it possible to make up for the disruption of other peripheral meridians. Although other meridian lines can be involved in the first signs of fatigue, it is essential to ensure the circulation of meridians 33 and 34 as well as 35 and 37 for women and 36 and 38 for men. This will strengthen overall spatial orientation and sharpen motor coordination, while granting awareness of personal boundaries in the surrounding space.

EXPRESSING OUR COGNITIVE IDENTITY AS A MAN OR WOMAN

Being centered, consistent, and present to oneself and others is not always easy! Even if we wish to be in "top form," we can sometimes fall victim to reflex reactions, habits, and emotions that gain the upper hand over our mental capabilities. And if, thanks to experience, our cerebral cortex transforms and permanently reorganizes its elements, it can often play tricks on us.

Indeed, how much information must we filter simultaneously to interact with our environment, make decisions, and make choices? Drowning in a swamp of data to select, most of our responses are often automatic for lack of time and sometimes want of deliberation. Today, in a milieu saturated by all kinds of stimulations, we often have trouble remaining vertical or taking a step backward; we get dragged into spirals of hyperactivity, which throw the discernment and awareness that should be guiding us off kilter. In Nutripuncture, this involves a loss of cerebral conduction, a "loss of identity," manifesting through various disorders (confusion, irritability, insomnia, asthenia, alienation, and so on), which can later degenerate into severe depression (or anger) and extensive somatic modifications.

As sociologist Alain Ehrenberg notes, the society of performance and success weakens individuals, inducing inability-to-act disorders and depressions linked to the feeling of not "being up to the challenge."[1] Self-mastery, mental flexibility, the ability to take action: everyone of us needs to be constantly adapting to an unstable and temporary world composed on moving trajectories.

Today it is crucial to support the performance ability of our cerebral cortex!

First and foremost it is essential to express the identity that characterizes each of us and the sensibility that makes each of us a unique and valuable individual. But it is also important to stimulate our creativity, give meaning to the choices we make, and most especially to achieve an important mission: to live in tune with our cognitive and sensory identity. This is certainly no simple task; it is a complex process that begins at birth and never ends.

In fact, our cognitive attitudes develop in accordance with our personal history, and through the experience that draws the neurological circuits that wire our cerebral cortex. Flexible and changing, the connections between neurons are constantly reshaping themselves, transforming our sensibilities and the way we look at things. However, while the most amazing quality of the cortex is its plasticity, a number of parameters can interfere with the dynamics of this incredible "control tower" of the body. Furthermore, the cortex is the headquarters for cognitive memory, a great human wealth that we each should protect to counter oblivion. Reinforcing its potential is therefore essential!

Just What Is Identity?

In Nutripuncture, identity forms a fundamental parameter that shapes the psychophysical balance of human beings, always considered as inseparable from their context and network of relationships, which is what makes it possible for identity to exist and transform. This vital context, in which nothing is separate but where everything communicates, is in reality formed by differentiated elements that interact without stop, recognizing their uniqueness and enriching themselves through the mutual exchange of their differences.

While there does exist an elementary reference frame on the biological level, defined for example by unique finger prints, the research undertaken by Nutripuncture practitioners has shown this basic reference frame is a code that calls on all systems of the organism, a kind of "identity signature" that coordinates cellular life, ensures its integrity, and orchestrates its coherent expression. The hypothesis has been ventured that it may be a kind of sensory core, containing initial foundational elements that shape the particular sensibility of every individual. In fact, if identity manifests on the genetic, constitutional level through the shapes that characterize the unique morphology of an individual (shape of the ears, nose, the iris, and so on), it also expresses itself through parameters of an informational

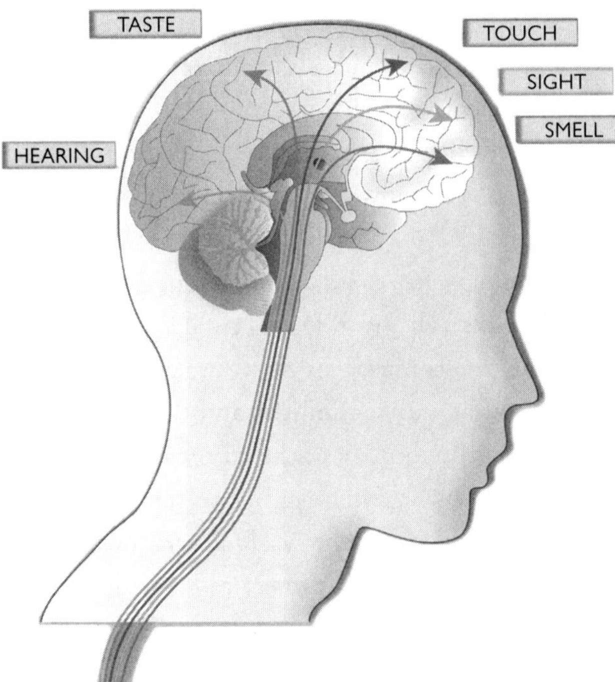

Fig. 3.17. Our senses, and, thus, the way we experience the world, are key factors in identity.

nature, such as the timbre of a person's voice or his or her particular perception (fig. 3.17; see also color insert).

Although identity represents a fundamental ingredient of our vitality, it is simply an essential frame of reference for expressing our uniqueness while recognizing and respecting the uniqueness of the other, without any fusion or confusion! Our organs also have a distinctive identity: my liver, for example, is not like that of my neighbor! The information it has recorded through my entire life is completely unique: my energy, the things that make me mad, my diet, and so forth, have all colored its functioning and shaped its vitality. Its relations with the other organs, their dynamic interactions, have also played a part in making my liver the only one of its kind in the world. Not to mention the identity codes (DNA) that give it its character, as well as its polarity (male or female). Each organ, just like every cell of the body, keeps in its memory the XX or XY sex codes that characterize an individual.

To encourage the expression of our cognitive potential and awaken our ability to think deeply, Nutripuncture offers stimulation to the meridians that ensures the high performance level of the body's control tower:

Meridian line 08, cognitive integration
Meridian line 12, shaping instinct, hormonal equilibrium, and emotional balance
Meridian line 02, involved in postural balance, and therefore verticality
Meridian line 26, ensuring motor conduction

Obviously, when you are dealing with these areas, you are also dealing with the central nervous system, which will be more effectively regulated if the other vital parameters are already in their proper places—that is, if you are present in the here and now (meridian lines 27 and 28 for women; meridian lines 21 and 27 for men) and your sensory perception has been stimulated and your spatial orientation is correctly positioned (meridian lines 33 and 34). This underscores the importance of gradually stimulating all of the factors that influence our vitality, depending on their roles, from the most basic to the more complex.

Here, in broad lines, are the ingredients that play a role in maintaining our vitality at an optimum level and the meridian lines we recommend supporting first to ensure the best overall dynamics. Whether a person is a child, an adult, or elderly, or an athlete seeking to enhance his performance and particular presence, these parameters need to be maintained on a regular basis because they are constantly being challenged by our daily lives.

But this is only the beginning! We are continuing to seek in our body's complexity for the parameters that are responsible for other more subtle performance levels, such as creativity, for example, or visual projection, in order to better understand our body's language and the information that stimulates or inhibits its dynamics and evolution.

4
Sensory Personality Types

UNDERSTANDING THE MECHANISMS of the body's cybernetics, which link organic functions together as support for human behavior, is a challenge that is still far from having been met. However, for several thousand years, Asian acupuncturists have been able to describe the relationships between the body and the mind in terms of the body's communication circuits. These are the meridians, which shape our behavior without our knowing.

While traditional acupuncture relates the meridians to the five elements of traditional Chinese medicine—Earth, Water, Metal, Fire, and Wood—Nutripuncture relates them to the five elements of Ayurvedic (Traditional Indian) medicine and traditional Tibetan medicine—Earth, Water, Air, Fire, and Ether. With regard to Ether, Nutripuncture prefers to use the term *Boundary* or *Limit* because it corresponds to the sense of touch (skin). Each of the other elements also corresponds to one of the five sensory faculties:

Earth — Taste

Water — Hearing

Air — Smell

Fire — Sight

Ether — Touch

FIVE SENSES FOR PERCEIVING THE WORLD AND BUILDING OURSELVES

Our five types of perception are communicational modalities, which reveal the sensory and relational acuity of every individual.

Taste, for appreciating and savoring life
Hearing, for listening and learning to communicate
Smell, for experiencing the complete essence
Vision, for recognizing and illuminating
Touch, for establishing contacts

Sensory perception is an act of recognition—of re-knowing—a process allowing us to identify a piece of information (gustatory, sonorous, odorous, visual, or tactile) and situate it within the surrounding space. Thanks to this five-path sensibility, fed by the thirty-three meridians, we can distinguish and work out the sensations flowing from our perception in order to build an immense data bank, individually specific, our memories. But this only works when our senses are interactive and animated by cooperation and mutual recognition. This again depends on the harmonious circulation of the vital currents that feed our senses.

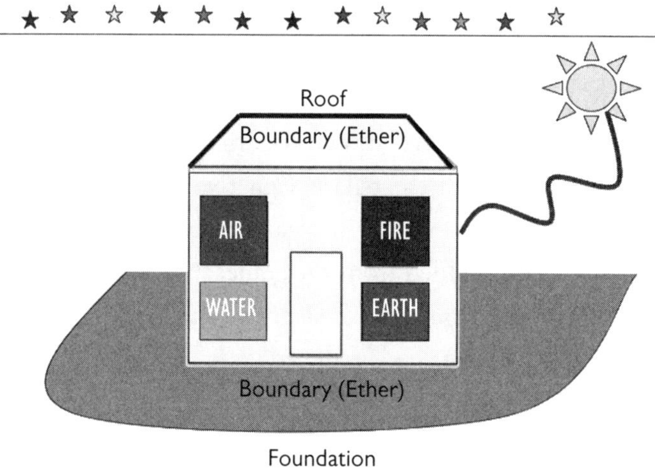

Fig. 4.1. The body is like a house.

Meridians and Sensory Perception

Each meridian family has a relationship with one of the five senses, whose performance it governs.

The Kidneys/Bladder pair modulates the sense of hearing, related to the element Water. These meridians ensure hearing, tuning in to yourself and others.

The Stomach/Spleen-Pancreas pair feeds the sense of taste, related to the element Earth. These meridians nurture the capacity for enjoying life and savoring material reality.

The Lungs/Colon pair regulates the sense of smell, related to the element Air. These meridians feed our instincts and ensure the awakening of our feelings.

The Heart/Small Intestine pair governs the sense of sight that is activated by light and is related to the element Fire. This pair directs the projection of sight, making it possible to illuminate reality in accordance with our cognitive maturity.

The joint activity of the Liver/Gall Bladder and Master of the Heart/Triple warmer pairs governs touch and the ability to establish contact both physically and emphatically. These two centers of regulation are related to the element Ether (boundary or limit).

Normally our sense receptors work together simultaneously to provide us an overall and integrated perception of the surrounding reality. In this way, the information captured by each sense is combined with others and takes part in the decoding of all the nuances of the stimuli being perceived. For example, tasting a food stimulates our taste buds but it also stimulates our nose with its fragrance. At the same time, our eyes' attention is drawn to its shape and color, while its texture arouses the tactile sensibility of the palate. Our five senses jointly contribute to a single experience, which would not be as pleasant, full, and "nourishing" if one of the sensory receptors was excluded from the game, such as, for example, what happens when we are suffering from a cold. Without the active presence of our sense of smell, the sensitivity of our taste is reduced.

Our five senses, each with their own receptors and sensibility, are not isolated, but form a real team that allows us to simultaneously capture a large amount of different kinds of information. The dynamic of our five senses is a valuable legacy that allows us to situate ourselves within the natural and social context with which we interact. The ideal is to have a harmonious sensory dynamic shaping our vital currents and therefore our behavior.

Meridians in Balance

When our meridians are in balance, our senses function optimally. What follows is an outline of each sense, its related meridians, the role each meridian plays, and the resulting optimal performance.

Vision: Heart/Small Intestine Family (04/13)

Meridian line 04 (Heart): rhythm, desire, plan, enthusiasm, decision, ability to recognize, self-esteem, projective thought

Meridian line 13 (Small Intestine): choice, selection

Gaze: sharp, projective, piercing, warm, tender, revealing, luminous, benevolent, frank, determined

Combines with taste, hearing, smell, and touch

Taste: Stomach/Spleen-Pancreas Family (10/18)

Meridian line 10 (Stomach): taste for effort, ability to take action, will, courage, and respect for one's capacities

Meridian line 18 (Pancreas): transformation, making things concrete, realization of action, logical and concrete thought

Taste: structured, receptive, refined, measured, has discriminating palate

Combines with hearing, smell, sight, and touch

Hearing: Kidney/Bladder Family (22/31)

Meridian line 22 (Kidney): inner assurance, zest for life, contemplative thinking

Meridian line 31 (Bladder): alertness, objectivity

Listening qualities: profound, attentive, keen, true, selective

Combines with taste, smell, sight, and touch

Smell: Lungs/Colon Family (20/05)

Meridian line 20 (Lungs): confidence, creativity, personal inspiration, and expression of one's male or female individuality, imaginative and philosophical thought

Meridian line 05 (Colon): organization, ability to give orders, prioritizing tasks.

Sense of smell: have a good nose, feel all the subtleties of things
Combines with taste, hearing, sight, and touch

Touch: Liver/Gall Bladder Family (11/30) and the Master of the Heart (35/36) and Triple Warmer (37/38) Family

Meridian line 11 (Liver): wisdom, understanding
Meridian line 30 (Gall Bladder): serenity
Master of the Heart (35/36) and Triple Warmer (37/38): mastery, control, and consistency
Touch: revelatory, magnetic, sensitive, tactful, feeling comfortable in one's own skin
Combines with taste, hearing, smell, and sight

Meridians Out of Balance

Our research has revealed that in reality our overall perception is often inhibited by our attitudes and that some people only trust their taste buds, their nose, or what they can see, thereby fragmenting the overall sensory dynamic. This has several consequences, on both the sensory and behavioral level.

Human beings, unlike animals, are capable of interfering with their body's natural knowledge in order to adjust to social and cultural codes, which are not always respectful of the body's biological expression. We have observed that a kind of competition sometimes exists between our sensory receptors, which can disrupt the circulation of their corresponding meridians. For example, although humans often rely on sight more than smell (which is more developed in animals), some people have a conflict between visual and tactile perception, obliging them to shut their eyes in order to activate their cutaneous sensitivity more fully. These habits dull certain meridians because they place a constant demand upon them and isolate them from the active support of the other meridian lines. This causes a gradual diminishment of their vitality.

In this way, over the years, we drift further from knowledge of our own bodies by gradually anesthetizing our sensory finesse, which becomes increasingly crushed beneath the mind and abstract thoughts. We have trouble tuning in to our sensations; our gestures become mechanical and deliberate. Though they are efficient, they no longer have any meaning or humanity. We calculate, we measure, we seek to master everything, whereas the goal of the game is to learn through and from our experiences and sensations, to integrate them in order to gain self-knowledge, to grow and realize ourselves without forgetting "the senses" of life offered by our body.

SENSORY PERSONALITY TYPES: FRAGMENTED SENSORY DYNAMICS AND BEHAVIOR

We have seen that behind our five senses there are thirty-three vital currents that are ceaselessly working, modulating our behavior and relational attitudes. The hundreds of pieces of information recorded by our sensory receptors and adjusted by the vital currents circulate through the entire body and change into emotions and feelings. Based on emotional and relational circumstances, we express particular attitudes and activate various sensory personality types, showing the variability of our moods and the plasticity of our perceptions.

A *sensory personality type* is an individual predisposition, a terrain, which results from two interactive systems, the *innate* and the *acquired.* One is *constitutional:* it is our physique and our structure and is formed from the genes we have inherited from our genetic line. The other is *informational,* and is connected with our experience, our sensibility, and the way our inherited genetic potential is "managed." The countless pieces of information contained in these two systems modulate the body's self-regulation and ensure individual expression.

The first system is directly connected to parental heredity; it is the baggage we are born with. The second, on the other hand, is built out of our experiences and managed by the sensibility of each individual. It contains the information recorded during childhood and adjusted by education, the relations woven with our parents, the stimuli received from the environment, and so forth. This acquired system, resulting from our personal experience, plays a fundamental role in the projection of individual characteristics, which are necessary for the management of genetic memory and inherited family behavior patterns.

When the innate system with its genetic memories gains the upper hand, the individual's behavior will be imitative, similar to that of his parents or extended family. This is the well-known phenomenon of "familial mimetism." In the learning process, the child identifies with parental projections and adjusts his or her behavior to conform to their wishes. Later, as adults, we often unknowingly continue living in accordance with our mother's taste, our father's experience, our grandfather's view of things, in our grandmother's skin, instead of asserting our own sensory individuality, the heart of our identity. It is therefore important to sharpen our five senses in order to fully benefit from each of their particular sensibilities, which sometimes remain unexpressed.

Nutripuncture studies have made it possible to gain a better understanding of the close relationship between our five senses and the vital currents nourishing them, which give each of us our unique physical and mental sensibility. Specific profiles have been gradually identified, five "sensory personality types," which combine and interact with each other, revealing each person's perceptional habits and relational attitudes. Although all human beings manifest tendencies encapsulating these different personality types, over time the majority of us activate one of the five perceptive modalities more while inhibiting the others.

For example, there are people of a gustatory personality type for whom taste is a fundamental structuring and dynamizing perception—in short, an essential benchmark used as the ultimate reference. They are very active individuals with a determined go-getter attitude, who can often be hyperactive. In this same personality type we also find individuals who are slothful and lazy, who are sometimes anorexic, who have lost their zest for life and any taste for working or desire to express themselves. These individuals totally neglect their gustatory perception.

Taste and Its Four Receptors

Our taste buds possess four kinds of different receptors: bitter, sweet, acidic, and salty, permitting us to appreciate these flavors in accordance with our gustatory sensibility, broadly managed by the Stomach/Spleen-Pancreas family. The synergy of these four fundamental flavors becomes activated thanks to contact with the tongue and palate, from which the sense of the palatability of a food emanates. During our research, we saw that people who preferred or detested certain flavors, such as sweet or acidic, for example, displayed hyper- or hypo-activity of the corresponding receptors, in connection with the activity of certain meridian lines. This is why, when heavy demands are placed on the Kidneys/Bladder family, a person can adore (or become downright intolerant of) sweet foods, milk, cheese, and so forth. This demonstrates the interaction of the 22/31 pair (which modulates the sensitivity of the sweet flavor), with the 10/18 family (which adjusts the perception of bitter flavors more), an interaction that also takes place with the 04/13 family (salty flavor) and the 20/05 family (acidic flavor).

This example underscores the impact sensory perception has on our behavior, which it shapes without our knowing, and the importance of the overall sensory balance, which is a product of the harmonious interaction of the five senses. When each receptor plays its role interactively with the others, without any competition or inhibitions, our behavior also becomes harmonious. However it has been seen that as individuals grow older, most of us use a particular personality type more often, which thereby weakens some of our vital currents. Even though we might change behavior in accordance with our emotional state and relational context, the changes are usually between attitudes that are all associated with one personality type. For example, we might be shy with our lovers, authoritarian with our work colleagues, and sentimental with our parents.

Unbalanced Meridians and Dysfunctional Behaviors

When the meridians are unbalanced, dysfunctional behaviors can result. For each of the sensory personality types given below, a lack of balance can be due to either a weak or overly strong functioning of the related meridians.

Visual Personality Type: Sentimental Attitude

This personality type is a result of a weakened Heart/Small Intestine family (04/13). It is evidenced by a gaze that is blasé, dull, sleepy, murderous, hypnotic, greedy, or black.

When meridian line 04 is functioning too weakly, it induces:

- Emotional instability
- Lack of desire, no plans, no enthusiasm, no rhythm, being dominated by emotions
- Vital need to be loved and acknowledged by others (cannot acknowledge oneself)
- Devotion, sacrifice, life dedicated to others
- Kindness that alienates others, excessive solicitude
- Guilt feelings (for real or imagined wrongs)
- Feelings of worthlessness, self-deprecation
- Bending over backward for forgiveness
- Being a spendthrift, overly generous

When meridian line 04 is functioning too strongly, it induces:

Difficulty in sharing, egotism, avarice
Narcissism, vanity
Seduction, seeking to please, being a slick talker or charmer
Jealousy, being tempestuous or impetuous

When meridian line 13 is functioning too weakly, it induces:

Indecision, abulia (lack of will), irresolution, difficulty making choices
Submission to the choices made by others
Sensation of inner emptiness (saving things for fear of needing them later)

When meridian line 13 is functioning too strongly, it induces:

Determination to please others with no personal benefit
Being eaten up by the desire to compensate
Bulimic behavior from emotional emptiness

If there is any kind of excess or defect, stimulation of the Heart/Small Intestine family (see chapter 8), will prompt its self-regulation.

Stimulation of meridians 04 and 13 with Nutris will encourage:

The desire to give and share
The ability to make plans
The expression of one's deepest desires
Better understanding of oneself and others
Greater vital impetus and greater capacity to love
The freedom to make choices for oneself
Better visual projection, which will interact with the other senses

Gustatory Personality Type: Hyperactive and Authoritarian Attitude

This personality type is a result of a weakened Stomach/Spleen-Pancreas family (10/18). It is evidenced by taste that is greedy, voracious, gluttonous, and tasteless/lacking good taste.

When meridian line 18 is functioning too weakly, the individual:

Is dominated by work and his boss or superiors
Has difficulty making things a reality, structuring, changing
Is submissive and dutiful

When meridian line 18 is functioning too strongly, the individual:

Is excessively willful or logical

Lives only for work

Is scornful, ruthlessly ambitious (a social climber), dominating

Proud, pretentious, authoritarian

Is a man or woman of power, of learning, who is excessively rationalistic, wanting to prove everything and always be right

When meridian line 10 is functioning too weakly, it induces:

Difficulty taking action

Laziness, sloth, instability

Passivity, placidity, idleness

When meridian line 10 is functioning too strongly, it induces:

Forced action: the sense that "something must be done"

Hyperactivity, trying to do to much, getting overloaded

Wanting to do everything oneself, inability to delegate to others, impatience

If there is any kind of excess or defect, stimulation of the Stomach/Spleen-Pancreas family (see chapter 7), will prompt its self-regulation.

Stimulation of meridians 10 and 18 with Nutris will encourage:

Respect for one's potential for action and abilities to take action, change, and achieve

Acknowledgment of the work of others

Awareness of one's physical limitations with mastery of moderate effort

A sense of a job well done, a taste for effort, more stability, better material realization of plans

A voice that fits one's personality better, with more body

Better taste perception that is interactive with the other senses

Olfactory Personality Type: A Perfectionist and Idealist Temperament

This personality type is a result of a weakened Lungs/Colon family (20/05). It is evidenced by a sense of smell that is hyper- or hypo-sensitive, off target, without flair, or absent (asnomia).

When meridian line 20 is functioning too weakly, it encourages:

Domination by a familial, professional, social, political, or religious ideology
Gulliblity, naïvete
Being a devotee of an ideology, idol, politician, or guru
Fear of deceiving others, easily fooled by others (tendency to idealize them)
Seeking a model, wanting to resemble this individual, to be like that person
Living for one's image, being a follower of trends and fashions, without originality or imagination
Feeling unworthy, often confused, shame
Lacking hope and trust, with no faith in oneself (and seeking to place it in others)
Defeatism, pessimism
Disillusionment, disenchantment
Nostalgia, melancholy

When meridian line 20 is functioning too strongly, the individual is:

Fanatic, extremist, exalted (guru, leader of an ideology)
Convinced he or she is the keeper of the truth, proselytizer
Intolerant, intransigent, sectarian, doctrinaire
Conformist, takes everything literally

When meridian line 05 is functioning too weakly, it results in:

Total lack of rigor and organization
Disorganization, anarchy

When meridian line 05 is functioning too strongly, the individual is:

Tense, tight, obsessive, not flexible
Rigid, stiff
Formal, affected, haughty
Perfectionist
Fussy, cranky, puritanical
A stickler for things

If there is any kind of excess or defect, stimulation of the Lungs/Colon family (see chapter 8) will prompt its self-regulation.

Feeding meridians 20 and 05 with Nutris will encourage:

Self-confidence, deeper and more authentic inspiration
Optimal organization of work and other activities
Acknowledgement of the aspirations of others without judgment
More tolerance of self and others
A better olfactory perception that is interactive with the other senses

Auditory Personality Type: Timid and Fearful Attitude

This personality type is a result of a weakened Kidneys/Bladder family (22/31). It results in being hard of hearing (off key), auditory hallucinations, and so on.

When meridian line 22 is functioning too weakly, it induces:

Anguish, anxiety
Timidity, muteness, difficulty hearing
Lack of assurance
Fear of the future, fear of getting old
Fear of hurting oneself or causing harm to others
Fear of death, of life, of sexuality, emptiness, cold, or water
Being dominated by fears and worries
Being withdrawn, inhibited, self-effacing
All phobias (claustrophobia, agoraphobia, and so on)

When meridian line 22 is functioning too strongly, it induces:

Fear of nothing, daredevilry
Bravado in the face of danger
Recklessness

When meridian line 31 is functioning too weakly, it induces:

Lack of alertness, confusion
Pretending to see nothing, to know nothing, preference to remain unaware

When meridian line 31 is functioning too strongly, it induces:

Illusion, blindness, wanting to see the world through rose-colored glasses
Letting the wool be pulled over one's eyes, hallucinations

If there is any kind of excess or defect, stimulation of the Kidneys/Bladder family (see chapter 7) will prompt its self-regulation.

Feeding meridians 22 and 31 with Nutris will encourage:

More assurance and objectivity
More alertness in the courses of action taken
More facility expressing one's point of view, without fear
Reduction of timidity
Objective risk assessment
Better communication with others
The ability to tune in more deeply and extensively

Tactile Personality Type: Aggressive-Apathetic Attitude

If imbalance of these four personality types persists for a long period of time, it can impact tactile perception and the balance of the metabolic and cerebral poles, resulting in either an overly aggressive attitude—if the Liver/Gall Bladder family (11/30) is weakened—or an apathetic attitude—if the Master of the Heart/Triple Warmer family (35/36 and 37/38) is weakened. In either case the touch becomes vulgar, disrespectful, insensitive, clinging, invasive, and clammy.

When meridian line 11 is functioning too weakly, it encourages:

A taciturn personality, often depressive and beset with dark moods
Self-destructive tendencies, suicidal
Domination by bad moods
Often being cross with oneself

When meridian line 11 is functioning too strongly, it encourages:

Raging over trifles, losing temper easily, irritableness
Impulsiveness, being excessive or immoderate
Sarcasm, being scathing and unruly
Aggression, quarrelsomeness, being mad at everyone
Liking to pick fights, being brutal, violent

When meridian line 30 is functioning too weakly, the individual is:

Irritable, worrying a lot
Resentful, embittered

When meridian line 30 is functioning too strongly, the individual is:

Spiteful, cantankerous, bitchy, grumpy, complaining
Surly, off-putting, acerbic

If there is any kind of excess or defect, stimulation of the Liver/Gall Bladder family (see chapter 7) will prompt its self-regulation.

Feeding meridians 11 and 30 with Nutris will encourage:

Impulse-control, less anger
The ability to forgive oneself
More calm and tranquillity
The power required for an action
Dietary moderation
More delicate tactile sensitivity, combined with the other senses

When meridians 35/36 and 37/38 are functioning too weakly, that results in:

Depressive tendencies
Indolence, indifference, lack of vigor and vitality
Insensitivity, inertia, despondency
Lack of nerve force (physical magnetism)

When meridians 35/36 and 37/38 are functioning too strongly, that results in:

Excess of nervous energy
Very intense intellectual life
Lack of contact with the concrete reality of life

If there is any kind of excess or defect, stimulation of the Master of the Heart/Triple Warmer family (see chapter 8) will prompt its self-regulation.

Feeding meridians 35/36 and 37/38 with Nutris will encourage:

The sensation of feeling comfortable in one's own skin
A more harmonious presence with oneself and others
More consistency in life
Awareness of one's own limits and those of others
More physical and intellectual vitality
The expression of one's male or female sensibility
A more rewarding tactile perception, combined with the other senses

REGENERATION, NOT DEGENERATION

How would we cope without our five senses? These valuable "physical tools" are life instruments that make it possible to perceive outside reality and at the same time express our inner sensibility. Although many factors can weaken the vitality of our perceptions, we often grant little attention to a drop in our sense of smell or hearing, or the first signs of visual or gustatory problems. We consider them as inevitable, a normal consequence of our life style and the aging process.

In Nutripuncture, however, we regard these as valuable signals that need to be heeded, witnesses to the poor management of our own resources, heralding the premature weakening of the vital currents. "Everything that is not regenerating is degenerating," Edgar Morin likes to say, invoking a biological law that is valid for everything, for nothing should ever be taken for granted. To avoid deluding ourselves and to restore full sensibility, it is essential to support the performance of our five senses that are sometimes thrown out of whack by bad habits or by experiences we are not able to "digest," "feel," "see," "hear," and so forth, and which congest the circulation of our vital currents. Sharpening the sensitivity of our senses and supporting their interaction, in addition to ensuring an active, awake, and delicate perception, encourages better communication with ourselves and others. This is one of the main objectives of Nutripuncture.

5
Maintaining Vitality through Every Season of the Year

A SIMPLE BUT STATE-OF-THE-ART method for kicking off the work of awakening and gradually honing sensory perception consists of attuning the dynamics of the vital currents to the rhythm of the seasons.

Depending on our personal personality type, we can feel an affinity to one season more than the others. In the West, some people prefer one season to the others because they feel their best during that period of the year. On the other hand, they notice a decline in vitality during certain seasons—for example, an aggravation of lung disorders in autumn, or a recurrence of lumbar pains in winter. Nutripuncture offers an excellent way to keep our biorhythms in balance. It can be used to support and reinforce the vital currents used during each season, to ensure their vitality throughout the entire year, and to avoid the seasonal irritants that appear regularly and with greater intensity every year as we grow older.

This maintenance application of Nutripuncture can be begun at any time during the year, no matter what season it is. To get the best advantage from the rising energy in the meridians concerned, it is better to start at the beginning of the season and continue for three weeks or more, depending on the level of the vitality of the meridians you wish to support.

NUTRIPUNCTURE IN SUMMER: SHARPENING YOUR SIGHT

This is the time of the year when the sun reaches its zenith. Thanks to the intensity of its light, differences are revealed and details that are invisible in the dull light of winter can appear. Summer is related to the element of Fire, which gives light and heat: it is the season of desires and the time when projects are launched. Summer is the time to look at yourself and others in a new light in order to restore self-esteem and your desire to live, as well as to look at reality from a new perspective.

Depending on individual sensitivities, each person experiences summer differently. This season brings energy and a sense of well-being to some people. Others, in contrast, receive recurrent seasonal disorders that seem to get worse every succeeding summer as revealed by a lessened vitality. These disorders can include heart and circulation problems, disruptions of lipid metabolism and intestinal reabsorption, photosensitivity, and so forth. These problems can also be accompanied by hyperemotional and indecisive behavior, truly an inability to make choices.

The Heart/Small Intestine family presides over the development of the cerebral cortex, the part of the brain that determines individual character and allows the human being to attain self-awareness. This family therefore presides over the human psychological and intellectual development that follows on the heels of the metabolic maturation of early childhood. In fact, the goal of every evolutionary phase is to gain access to the potential of the central nervous system: its plasticity makes it possible to integrate one's experiences and benefit from them, and to refine one's sensibility by virtue of an increasingly effective neurological organization. Under these conditions life takes on all its sense, or rather its senses.

When meridian line 04 enables the Heart to assume its role as a projector and, on the psychological level, to express the desire "to be," meridian line 13 allows the Small Intestine to play its role in recognition and choice in reabsorbing the elements the best adapted for its metabolism.

With respect to this family's secondary meridians, meridian line 32 (Vision) will be at the height of its activity. This meridian line ensures the projection of one's gaze and outlook in synergy with meridian line 23 (Retina), which governs image reception. The activity of these two meridian lines is synergic: they should therefore be jointly stimulated in order to sharpen visual perception.

In Practice

You can take advantage of this time of year to strengthen the most sensitive meridian lines. This is the ideal moment for sharpening your sense of sight and vision by stimulating meridian line 32 (Vision) and 23 (Retina).

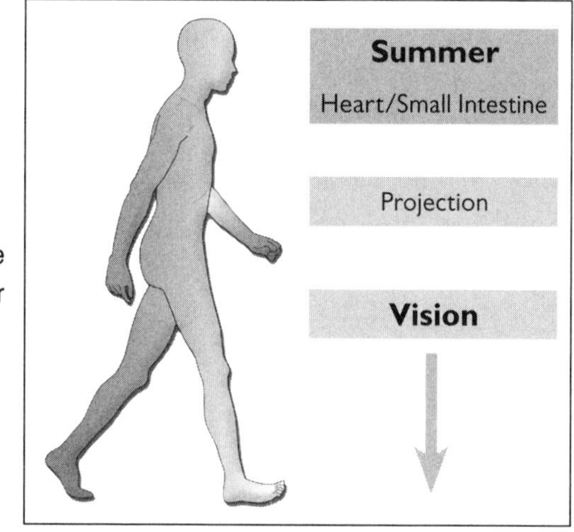

Fig. 5.1. Nutripuncture in summer

Sight and the Vital Currents of Summer

This is the time when the meridians of the Heart/Small Intestine family, particularly involved in the expression of feeling, need to be stimulated: meridian line 04, which shapes rhythm, and meridian line 13, which governs choice.

A lot of demands are also being made on secondary meridian lines of this family at this time, and they, too, require stimulation:

- Meridian line 01 of the Arteries, which expresses talent
- Meridian line 08 of the Cerebral Cortex, which governs cognitive integration
- Meridian line 32 of Sight, which activates the act of looking and hones your vision

NUTRIPUNCTURE FOR LATE SUMMER AND THE SEASONAL CUSPS: REFINING YOUR TASTE

According to Eastern tradition, between each of the four seasons there is a fundamental transitional period called the "*hwan* function." It is the return to Earth that demands the increased activity of the Stomach/Spleen-Pancreas family, which is producing its maximum energy output to manage the transition from one season to the next. For a period of around fifteen days, it forms a kind of interface between the season that is ending and the one just beginning. During the last week of the old season and the first week of the new one, the Stomach/Spleen-Pancreas meridians store the energy they've received from the "departing" family in order to gradually invest it in the family coming onto the stage.

After the potency of summer's Fire, the passage into action, overseen by the Stomach/Spleen-Pancreas family, proves to be of fundamental importance for achieving our plans hatched in the light of the Heart/Small Intestine family. Influenced by the gravitational charge of the element Earth, the Stomach/Spleen-Pancreas family governs anchoring in life. It allows us to set down roots, to have a certain "weight," and to be well-centered. The Earth element is primordial and essential; it is the densest of all elements and evokes the notion of the body. This family of meridian lines makes it possible to construct the essential reference points required for personality development. It governs the most mineral-like elements of the organism, the skeleton in particular, whose balance is connected with gravity.

Meridian line 10 of the Stomach is the vector of concrete action, the motor element of engendering life. It ensures sufficient strength on both the physical and psychological levels. On the digestive plane, it has an effect on the mouth cavity and stomach function. It provides these sectors all the power for their activities. The vital currents of the Stomach/Spleen-Pancreas family regulate the sense of taste: the taste for action, for undertaking new projects, for engendering, for creating life, and so on. Our relationship to our body is expressed through our sense of taste and this is at the heart of a number of behavioral disorders. Many problems that occur in puberty are the result of a conflict with one's body. The most important forms of stress (grief, suicide, divorce, abortion) can interfere with the psychosomatic dynamic and are always calling on the relationship maintained with the body.

This family adjusts the centripetal forces of the body in connection with specific secondary meridian lines: meridian line 17 (Bone) and 28 or 21 (Uterus or Prostate). We are therefore able take advantage of this season, as well as every seasonal cusp, to strengthen our bone and muscle system and invigorate our structural forces.

In Practice

The end of summer, like the other between season periods, is a crucial passage, as it calls on a very deep reference: one's body. During each "inter-season" you can jointly stimulate meridian line 10 (Stomach) and meridian line 18 (Pancreas) to "get your feet back on the ground," and activate all your potential for action. You can also take advantage of this season to rejuvenate the structural meridians that are often affected by all the annoyances in action, such as meridian line 28 (Uterus) for women and meridian line 21 (Prostate) for men.

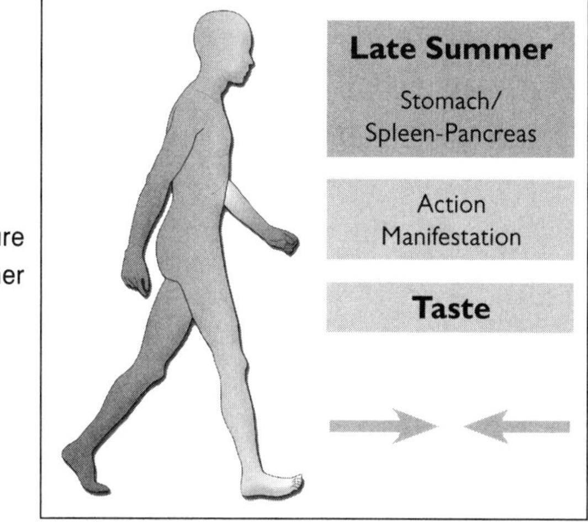

Fig. 5.2. Nutripuncture in late summer

Taste and the Vital Currents of Late Summer

Late summer (and similarly, each seasonal cusp) is defined by concrete action of the Stomach/Spleen-Pancreas family, ruler of this season, which enables the expression of our zest to exist, to enjoy life, to fit in, to take action, to change, and so on. The meridians experiencing the heaviest demands at this time are number 10, which shapes action, and 18, which governs transformation.

All the secondary meridian lines of this family are:

- Meridian line 17 of Bone, which governs the forces of structuring
- Meridian line 21 of the Prostate, which governs anchoring and realization for men
- Meridian line 26 of the Thalamus, which governs motor conduction
- Meridian line 28 of the Uterus, which governs anchoring and realization for women

Among them, it is particularly important to stimulate meridian line 28 of the Uterus for women and meridian line 21 of the Prostate for men to sharpen the sense of taste.

NUTRIPUNCTURE IN AUTUMN: REFINING YOUR SENSE OF SMELL

The passage of autumn is characterized by the activation of the vital currents of the Lungs/Colon pair, master meridian lines for this season. They make it possible for you to feel your full potential, to perceive its "effluvia" in order to organize your life in accordance with your inspiration and find all the subtleties offered you. It is the time to take a new breath, reorganize, and abandon conformity and rigidity, time to introduce more flexibility and openness into your life.

The meridians of this family permit men and women to express their personal sensibilities, their deep intuitions, and to discover a new impetus to get organized in accordance with their personal inspiration. Autumn is therefore an ideal time for drawing upon all the potential of your resources by encouraging the self-regulation of the vital currents and thereby benefiting from a new burst of energy.

In the case of an imbalance, these meridians can induce pulmonary weakness and colic, and can be exhibited psychologically by meticulous (or obsessive) behavior or, to the contrary, a tendency to sow disorder.

The Lungs and Colon meridians interact with the secondary meridian lines of this family. First among these are those that govern the rhinencephalic system (for which the hypothalamus is the orchestra conductor), related to the sense of smell. The olfactory system captures the information released by every part of the body. This information is a veritable distillate or essence of the body's cellular labors. Normally, the rhinencephalic system in human beings is under the control of the neo-cerebellum. It has been observed in Nutripuncture that this relationship is sometimes reversed: the rhinencephalon gains the upper hand over cerebral control. This inhibits the expression of individuality, and pushes the person toward a gregarious group identity and conformist attitudes, separating the individual from his or her own inspiration and feelings.

In a case like this, it is necessary to restore all its power to the sense of smell. This makes it possible to become aware of your uniqueness, to recognize and appreciate the unique fragrances of your own body, in short, to "wake up and smell the coffee" and become clued in about who you really are. For this, meridian line 25 (Sinus) and meridian line 12 (Hypothalamus) are stimulated in combination with the master meridians of this family: meridian line 20 (Lungs) and 05 (Colon).

The Lungs/Colon family plays a major role at the time of puberty, when the adolescent is in the midst of a complete transformation, and can have difficulties accepting these changes. In some cases refusal to accept this has been seen in a desire to be different or to resemble someone else. This transition can be helped along by stimulating meridian line 12, which governs the hormonal system, in combination with meridian line 24 for young women or meridian line 14 for young men.

The notion of sexual sensibility is a key one and ensures the expression of identity, the base for individual psychophysical equilibrium. If a need is felt to reinforce it, meridian lines 24 and 07 can be jointly stimulated for women, or meridian lines 14 and 06 for men. Breasts express the essence of female identity. The stimulation of meridian line 24 (Breasts) allows a woman to feel her femininity and fulfill her potential. This meridian line has a general effect on the odoriferous emanation of the upper half of the body (the sweat of the armpits). In contrast, meridian line 07 has much greater involvement in the odors released by the lower half of the body (inguinal perspiration). For men, meridian line 14 (Adam's Apple), which has quite a broad function like meridian line 24 for women, can be stimulated to invigorate masculine sensibility. In combination with meridian line 06 (Penis), it plays an essential role in the man's sex life and in the expression of his virility.

The Lungs/Colon family also plays an important role in the lymphatic system, and thus in the immune and hormonal systems. Meridian line 15 (Lymphatic Glands) transports all the information released by the body's metabolism and adjusts immune response.

For people experiencing muscle weakness, this is the time to stimulate meridian line 16 (Muscles) in order to recover greater flexibility and elasticity in both the physical and psychological planes.

In Practice

Autumn is the ideal time for joint stimulation of meridians 20 (Lungs) and 05 (Colon). This is the time, if you so desire, to give new impetus to your male or female sensibility by regulating the meridians that express it: meridians 24 and 07 for women or 14 and 06 for men.

This is also a good time for sharpening your sense of smell by invigorating the rhinencephalic system, governed by meridian line 12 (Hypothalamus) and meridian line 25 (Sinus).

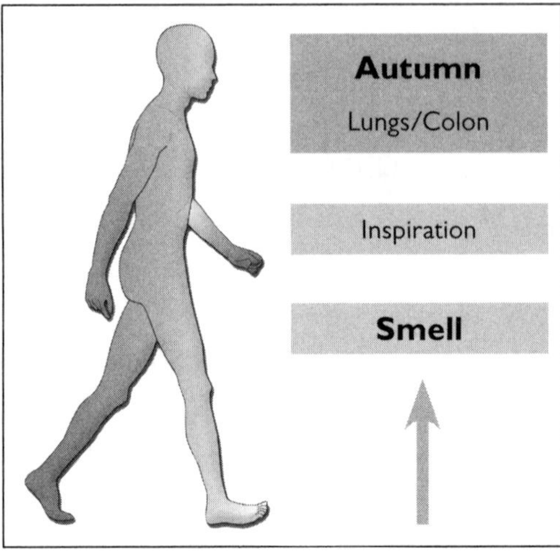

Fig. 5.3. Nutripuncture in autumn

Smell and the Vital Currents of Autumn

Autumn corresponds with the element of Air, which feeds the sense of smell. To encourage good respiratory dynamics and hone your sense of smell, it is important to help meridian line 20 of the Lungs, which governs breathing, to carry the vital breath to all the cells of the body. It is also essential to nourish meridian line 05 of the Colon, which regulates organization, to improve the elimination of metabolic wastes.

The secondary meridians of this family are:

- Meridian line 06 of the Penis, which regulates male sexuality
- Meridian line 07 of the Vagina, which regulates female sexuality
- Meridian line 12 of the Hypothalamus, which orchestrates the hormones and regulates instinct
- Meridian line 14 of the Adam's Apple, which expresses virility
- Meridian line 15 of the Lymphatic System, which regulates self-expression
- Meridian line 16 of the Muscles, which governs movement
- Meridian line 24 of the Breasts, which expresses femininity
- Meridian line 25 of the Sinus, which governs inspiration

Among them, meridian line 25 is the most important to stimulate for sharpening your sense of smell.

NUTRIPUNCTURE IN WINTER: SHARPENING YOUR HEARING

The psychophysical balance of this time of year is connected to the ability of the vital currents of the Kidneys/Bladder family to regulate their activities. In synergy with their secondary circuits, they govern the sense of hearing.

Some people find this time one that gives them energy and a sense of well-being. Others, in contrast, are prey to seasonal disorders, which gradually steal more vitality from their victims each year. These disorders include renal or vesical weaknesses, lumbar pains, disruption of venous circulation, and psychological disorders characterized by fears.

The pair of meridians 22 (Kidneys) and 31 (Bladder) preside over the formation of the embryo and correspond with an individual's genetic potential, the activation of which is dependent upon environmental stimuli. Based on genetically programmed biological constants, this pair controls the building of tissue in conformance with the original biological blueprint. It presides over genetic sexual transformation (XX or XY) in synergy with the secondary meridian lines. These include meridian line 09 (Adrenal Glands), which oversees the transmission of genetic potential, and meridian line 29 (Veins), which adjusts the returning information transported by the arteries. Meridian line 02 (Cerebellum) governs posture balance and muscle tone, in synergy with the inner ear. Meridian line 23 (Retina), in connection with image reception, is complementary to meridian line 32 (Vision), which oversees the attention of the gaze. Meridian line 27 (Thyroid) regulates the rhythm of our biological clocks. Winter is therefore the time to stimulate our resources through encouraging the self-regulation of the sectors that have been most weakened by this season, and thereby enjoy the benefits of a new burst of energy, This is the ideal time for invigorating the sense of hearing, and reinforcing posture and lumbar balance.

The invigoration of the Kidneys and Bladder meridians offers relaxation to fearful individuals who lack confidence, alertness, and who sometimes are living in a dream world. This stimulation can be very helpful for shy children.

In Practice

This is a season that invites introspection and assessing the past. It is therefore the time to provide support to the activity of meridian line 22 (Kidneys) and meridian line 31 (Bladder), support that can be essential when a person has reached an advanced age. This is the time to sharpen our hearing, especially if it has a tendency to become dull and lose its edge. Activating the Gonad meridians makes it possible to stimulate our confidence and better position our voice.

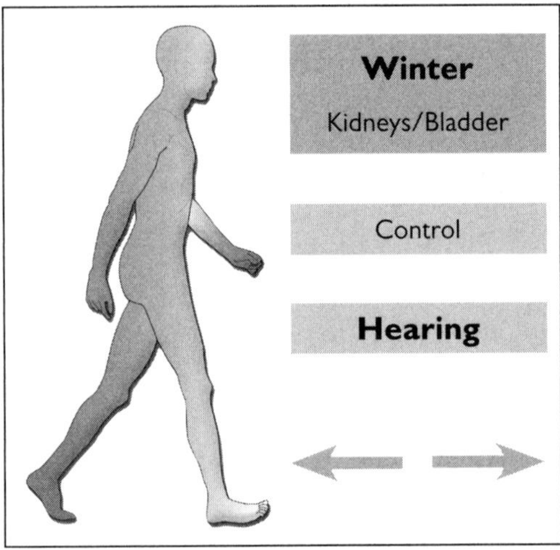

Fig. 5.4. Nutripuncture in winter

Hearing and the Vital Currents of Winter

Winter, linked with the element Water and the sense of hearing, encourages introspective work and enables you to tune in more clearly to yourself and others. Doing this kind of self-work allows you to see more clearly and reinforces your assurance and alertness, while dispelling your fears. In short, it makes it possible to achieve more authentic and lucid communication. In winter, it is therefore important to stimulate meridian line 22 (Kidneys), which governs assurance, and meridian line 31 (Bladder), which governs alertness and the communication of bodily fluids.

The secondary meridian lines of this family include:

- Meridian line 02 of the cerebellum, which governs postural balance
- Meridian line 09 of the Adrenal Glands, which provide source energy
- Meridian line 23 of the Retina, which shapes our depiction of reality
- Meridian line 27 of the Thyroid, which regulates time
- Meridian line 29 of the Veins, which governs receptivity

Among them, meridians 29 and 09 should particularly be given support to help sharpen your hearing.

NUTRIPUNCTURE IN THE SPRING: HONING YOUR SENSE OF TOUCH

Spring is the ideal time to turn over a new leaf and put on a new skin by providing support to the increased activity of the body's regulating currents: the meridians of the cerebral pole—governed by meridian lines 35 and 37 for women, and 36 and 38 for men—and the meridians of the metabolic pole—governed by meridian lines 11 and 30—which adjust for consistency the functioning of the vital current network. Our vitality at this time of year depends upon the harmonious interaction between these two centers. Working in synergy with other vital currents, these meridians play a role in the sense of touch.

The return to the source at the end of winter, a return to our own genetic memory: spring is experienced differently by everyone. For some, this period brings energy and a sense of well-being, for others, in contrast, it brings the return of seasonal disorders (hepatic weaknesses, apathy, fatigue), which reveal themselves

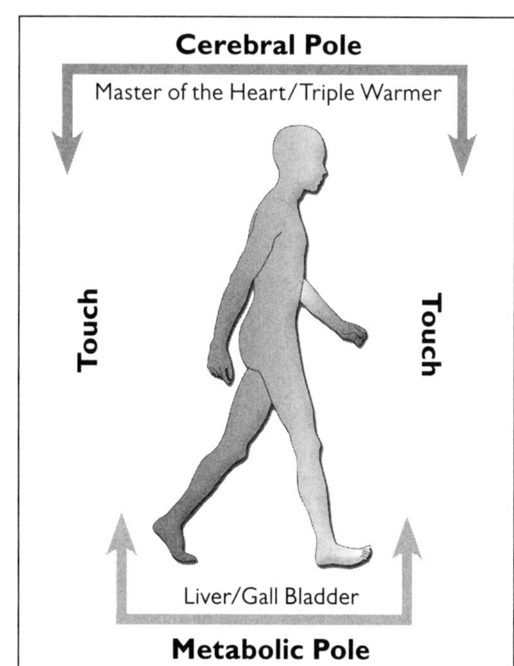

Fig. 5.5. Nutripuncture in spring

through a loss of vitality that worsens a little every passing year. These problems can also be accompanied by angry, even bitter behavior. Stimulation of meridian line 11 (Liver) and meridian line 30 (Gall Bladder) will allow people of an angry disposition to relax, as well as those who are overly aggressive or have a "bilious" personality lacking calm and tranquillity. Sometimes the joint regulation of the Master of the Heart meridians (35 female or 36 male) and Triple Warmer (37 female or 38 male), can help a person feel better in their own skin and face up to territorial conflicts and issues concerning personal space.

Touch and the Vital Currents of Spring

Spring is the season of renewal, when new sap rises in nature to launch a new cycle of life. It is related to the element Ether (Boundary or Limit). This is the time for us to shed our old skins in favor of the new and improve our sense of touch.

To support cellular renewal, it is important to nourish the meridians of the Liver/Gall Bladder family, so they may in turn supply our bodies with new energy. Meridian line 11 (Liver) influences metabolic activation and meridian line 30 (Gall Bladder) governs metabolic regulation. The activity of this family is adjusted by nerve meridians that shape the brain activity necessary to contain and limit metabolic activity:

- Meridian line 35 of the female Master of the Heart, cerebral activation
- Meridian line 36 of the male Master of the Heart, cerebral activation
- Meridian line 37 of the female Triple Warmer, cerebral regulation
- Meridian line 38 of the male Triple Warmer, cerebral regulation

The secondary meridians of this family are:

- Meridian line 03, expressing potency
- Meridian line 19, governing touch
- Meridian line 33 of Conception, which, with 34 of the Governor, governs spatial orientation
- Meridian line 34 of the Governor, which, with 33 of Conception, governs spatial orientation

Among them, support should especially be provided to meridian line 03 (Hair) and 19 (Skin) in order to sharpen the sense of touch.

PART TWO

Supporting the Meridians with Associative Nutripuncture

Vitality is a resource contained in the sensory and cognitive potential of every individual.

6
The Complexity of the Meridians

BEFORE WE EXPLORE the fairly complex dynamics and interactions of the thirty-eight meridians listed in Nutripuncture in depth, it will be helpful to take a short detour to better grasp the common denominators animating the countless expressions of life, among which our organism represents the most elaborate form.

TO EVERY KINGDOM ITS ELEMENT

In the complexity of life, everything is connected. As human beings we are connected to other beings phylogenetically: through the evolutionary development and diversification of groups of organisms. According to phylogenesis there is an order, a scale corresponding to the different levels of the appearance of life on Earth: the mineral, plant, animal, and, finally, the human (fig. 6.1). The human is the latest link in an incredible evolutionary chain, characterized by the interaction of the five elements, the essential components of life, each of which belongs to a given kingdom. In fact, the human body recapitulates the long evolution of life: from algae to mammals, it retains the memory of all the kingdoms that gave it birth.

The mineral kingdom. Thanks to the minerals attached to the protein-based framework, the densest element of life gives form to our skeleton. Minerals correspond with the element of Earth, related to the sense of taste, and are governed by the Stomach/Spleen-Pancreas family. These meridians preside over the development of part of the central nervous system, the thalamus (gray matter nuclei), which is the control center of our gestures.

The plant kingdom is related to the autonomic nervous system (also known as the vegetative system). It corresponds with the element of Water and is related to the sense of hearing and the Kidneys/Bladder family. These meridians preside over the development of part of the central nervous system, the cerebellum, which controls postural balance.

The animal kingdom corresponds to the organization of those organs whose interaction engenders complex organisms. This kingdom is characterized by the development of the rhinencephalon—the area of the forebrain in charge of the sense of smell, in connection with the Air element, controlled by the Lungs/Colon family. These meridians preside over the development of another part of the central nervous system, the hypothalamus, the control center for hormones and instinct.

Humans, last stage of this evolutionary chain, are symbolized by the Heart/Small Intestine family, which governs the development of the cerebral cortex. The development of the cerebral cortex is connected with the Fire element and the sense of sight. Humans are characterized by our level of consciousness, which enables us to project our thoughts and gaze upon the world and grasp all its subtleties.

The human is different from the other kingdoms due to the development of touch, which makes it possible for all people to achieve individuality limited by our

Kingdom	Element	Sense	Meridian
Human	Ether/Limit	Touch	Master of the Heart/Triple Warmer Liver/Gall Bladder
	Fire	Sight	Heart/Small Intestine
Animal	Air	Smell	Lungs/Colon
Plant	Water	Hearing	Kidneys/Bladder
Mineral	Earth	Taste	Stomach/Spleen-Pancreas

Fig. 6.1. According to phylogenesis there is an order, a scale corresponding to the different levels of the appearance of life on earth: the mineral, plant, animal, and, finally, the human, the latest link of this evolutionary hierarchy.

skin, characteristic of our psychological and spiritual uniqueness. This last element, Ether or Limit, is governed by the complementary activity of two families: Liver/Gall Bladder and Master of the Heart/Triple Warmer. On the cerebral level these meridians preside over the development of the meninges, three protective membranes that envelop our brain.

The Five Elements Essential to Life

The evolution of life out of simple elements occurred in stages, in accordance with a highly structured dynamic. To better define it, we can look at the growth of a plant. In the beginning all its potential is contained in a seed that requires Water to germinate and Earth for nourishment. It then emerges into the Air, seeks out the heat of the sun (Fire), and finally takes shape with boundaries (Ether) in accordance with its genetic programming. (See fig. 6.2.)

A similar though much more complex dynamic exists in humans. It calls on the same laws and elements: the sperm fertilizes the egg in the fallopian tube (Water), the egg then nestles in the uterus (Earth). On birth, we enter an atmospheric milieu (Air) with direct light (Fire), in order to grow and gradually draw our silhouette (Boundary/Ether), in accordance with the programming of our genes.

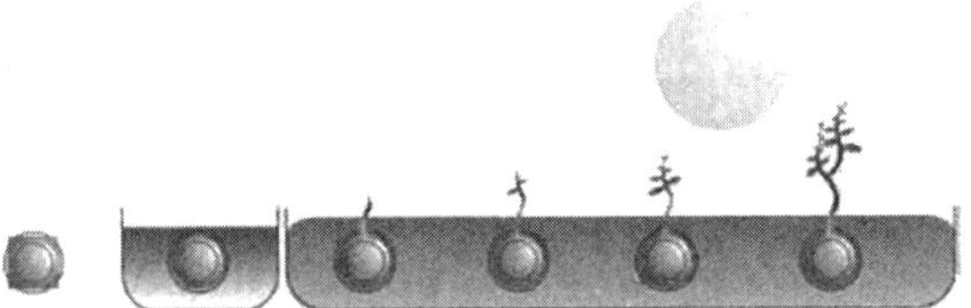

Fig. 6.2. The stages of plant growth, from the potential of the seed to full-grown plant

PERSONAL DEVELOPMENT

In the human being ontogenesis (the development of the individual organism from the earliest stage to maturity) proceeds differently than phylogenesis (the evolutionary development of the species). Ontogenetically, the fertilization of the ovum by the sperm occurs at the level of the element Earth, in connection with the Kidneys/Bladder family and its secondary meridians of the Gonads. Next the implantation of the egg and the construction of the body continues in the element of Earth in connection with the Stomach/Spleen-Pancreas family and its secondary meridian of the Uterus.

Conception and entering life are therefore ensured by the Kidneys/Bladder and the Stomach/Spleen-Pancreas families. A third family also plays a major role during the first phase of life construction, ensuring the energy necessary to maintain it. This is the Liver/Gall Bladder family, our energy center and the pole of metabolic regulation or "blood."

The activation of the rhythmic meridians of the upper half of the body occurs for the most part at puberty; they play a major role in the expression of sexual sensibility. The director of this evolutionary phase, a veritable transformation of the human being, is the Lungs/Colon family, which conducts the hormonal symphony. The relay is next picked up by the Heart/Small Intestine family, encouraging the cognitive maturation of the individual. For its part, the Master of the Heart/Triple Warmer family, the pole of neural regulation, shapes the expression of masculine or feminine individuality.

Meridians and Embryogenesis

While current research offers few answers regarding the induction of embryogenesis, there is general agreement regarding the existence of a preexisting order, a "boss" working as an internal clock, which guides the differentiation of the cells that will form the different tissues of the fetus.

The meridians can be considered as currents that transport the signals guiding cellular differentiation and that preside over the construction of the body. According to some researchers, they gradually appear in succession, thus creating the morphogenetic fields that will supply the framework on which the organs will form.

A FRAMEWORK OF FIVE FAMILIES

The consistency of organic complexity is orchestrated by the meridian network, which is divided into five families, each of which consists of two primary meridians, to which secondary meridians are connected. As mentioned earlier, Nutripuncture has assigned a number to each meridian line, in order to avoid confusing an organ with its meridian. Still, the families are referred to by the names of the significant organs to which the two primary meridians connect, much in the same way a highway can be named by a number or by the cities it crosses.

The meridians provide a kind of framework that connects all the sectors of the body and facilitates the communication between the individual and his or her environment. Nutripuncture research has explored each meridian in depth—in accordance with its role and its impact on individual psychophysical dynamics. Any disruption of a circuit (localized or chronic) can have an impact on the overall coherency of the network and thus cellular vitality.

PRACTICAL READING: HOW TO SUPPORT OUR MERIDIANS

In the two chapters that follow, we describe the role of each meridian as well as its interaction with the other vital currents of the body. Here you will also find listed the physical or mental conditions for which supporting the dynamics of one or more meridians lines with Associative Nutripuncture would be advisable. In every case, Associative Nutripuncture is preceded by the General Cellular Nutritional Regulator, Nutri Yin–Nutri Yang (also known as Liprofase in Italy). Then the Nutri corresponding to the particular meridian (with the same number) is taken, along with any other meridians that are listed. For example, in the description of meridian 22 on pages 94–95, "morning sickness" is connected with meridians 28 and 24, leading to a protocol of Nutri Yin–Nutri Yang + Nutri 22 + Nutri 28 + Nutri 24.

Chapter 7 details the metabolic meridians associated with the body's lower half and chapter 8 details the rhythmic meridians associated with the body's upper half.

A summary of the five families of the meridians and the roles and key words associated with each can be found on page 136.

7
The Metabolic Meridians of the Lower Body

WE BEGIN WITH THE MERIDIANS traveling through the body's lower half. They are the more metabolic families—Kidneys/Bladder, Stomach/Spleen-Pancreas, and Liver/Gall Bladder—which are very active from conception to adolescence.

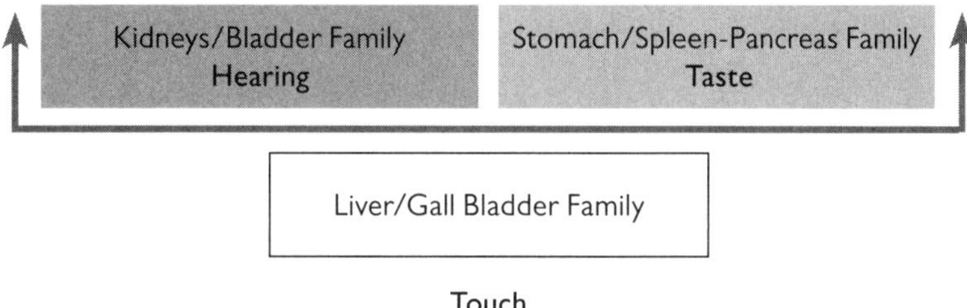

Fig. 7.1. The metabolic meridians of the lower body

KIDNEYS/BLADDER FAMILY—WATER ELEMENT—HEARING

The principal meridian lines of this family are 22 (Kidneys) and 31 (Bladder), combined with the secondary meridian lines 02 (Cerebellum), 09 (Suprarenal Glands), 23 (Retina), 27 (Thyroid), and 29 (Veins). This family regulates hearing, which presides over the acquisition of language and the expression of the body's sonorous potential. It is more sensitive in the winter.

This family manages the expression of genetic potential and controls the biological constants of the human body, shaping its centrifugal forces. While the Stomach/Spleen-Pancreas family governs the construction and the manifestation of the body, the Kidneys/Bladder family controls the transmission of innate information inherited through the genes, which is necessary for organic life.

The joint action of the secondary meridian lines 09 and 29 ensures the necessary gonadal activity for procreation.

Meridian line 27 marks time and facilitates the individual's coordination with life's various stages.

Meridian line 02 governs postural balance, while meridian line 23 ensures the equilibrium of visual representation. Each of these meridians also controls our mental and behavioral dynamics.

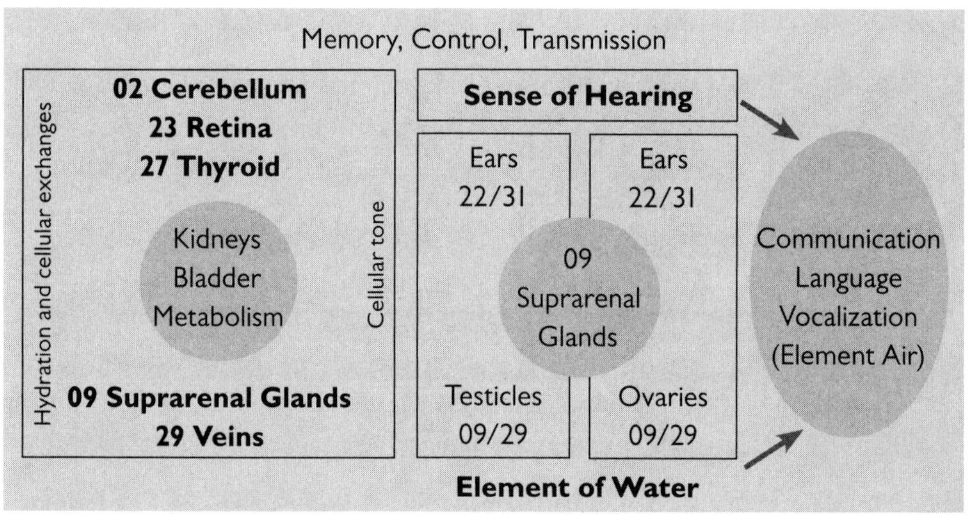

Fig. 7.2. Kidneys/Bladder Family: meridian lines 22 and 31

Meridian Line 22 of Assurance

Balances the Vital Currents of the Kidneys

Meridian line 22 constitutes the genetic reference frame. It manages hydrous balance and liquid exchanges at all tissue levels. It governs the maintenance of the biological constants. For this reason, this meridian line evokes inner assurance at the mental level, source of the popular French saying "to have solid kidneys" (whose figurative meaning is "to be in good financial shape").

Stimulating This Meridian Line Improves the Biological Terrain in the Following Cases

In a psychological context:

all fears (of death, getting pregnant, water, dark, loneliness, aging, and so on)
for a dentist visit or right before a surgical procedure
all phobias (agoraphobia, claustrophobia, and so on)
anxiety, stress
shy character, withdrawn, apprehensive (lack of assurance, not daring enough, blushes easily, and so on)
clumsy silence
for better integration with winter, combine with stimulation to meridian line 31

In a physical context:

urinary pathologies:
 for a woman, with meridian lines 33, 37, and 31
 for a man, with meridian lines 33, 38, and 31
to regulate blood pressure, with meridian lines 01, 04, and 29
dizzy spells and loss of balance, with meridian lines 02 and 31
nausea associated with morning sickness, with meridian lines 28 and 24
dehydrated skin, with meridian line 19
stiffness of the spinal column, excessive osseous thickening, combine with meridian lines 17 and 31

Meridian Line 31 of Alertness

Balances the Vital Currents of the Bladder

Meridian line 31 (Bladder) is a kind of mirror, well known to acupuncturists, which reflects the organs and their functions. On its pathway are the back *shu* points or "approvals," which reflect how efficiently the organs are operating. It is very long (starting on the internal edge of the eye and ending at the external edge of the fifth toe) and consists of a succession of sixty-seven points.

This is the meridian of alertness and reflection, prompting the objectivity necessary for grasping reality. The demands made upon this line are most heavy in winter.

Stimulating This Meridian Line Improves the Biological Terrain in the Following Cases

In a psychological context:

- lack of objectivity, clarity, alertness
- all fears, anxiety, timidity, with meridian line 22
- for better coping with the winter, with meridian line 22

In a physical context:

- urinary problems:
  - for a woman, with meridian lines 22, 37, and 33
  - for a man, with meridian lines 22, 38, and 33
- dizzy spell and loss of balance, with meridian lines 02 and 22
- stiffness of the spinal column, excessive osseous thickening, with meridian lines 17 and 22

Meridian Line 02 of Balance

Balances the Vital Currents of the Cerebellum

This meridian line controls the Water element on the level of the central nervous system. It thus ensures general and postural stability in relation to meridian lines 22 and 31. The Cerebellum, family tree of our ancestors' past lives, controls upright standing balance in relation to the inner ear. It controls the postural tonicity of rest, as well as voluntary and semi-voluntary motility. This meridian line plays the role of a pendulum, ensuring the harmonious interaction of the body's structural forces.

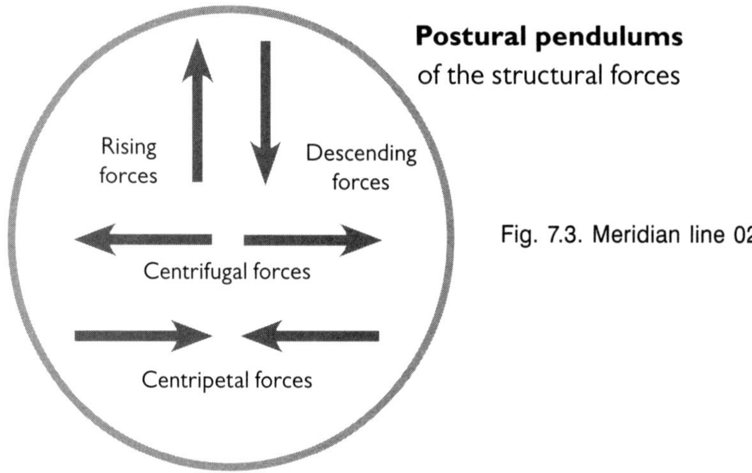

Fig. 7.3. Meridian line 02

Stimulating This Meridian Line Improves the Biological Terrain in the Following Cases

In a psychological context:

destabilization:

as a side-effect, with meridian line 04

from fear, with meridian line 22

In a physical context:

dizzy spell and loss of balance, with meridian lines 22 and 31

loss of sensitivity:

for a woman, with 35 and 37

for a man, with 36 and 38

for optimal muscular dynamics and fast recovery, the athlete can add meridian lines 08, 12, and 16

Meridian Line 09, Source

Balances the Vital Currents of the Adrenal Glands

By regulating the secretion rate of certain hormones, meridian line 09 (Suprarenal Glands) brings the necessary tonicity for fitting in to life. It is connected to postural balance, centered on the navel, which corresponds to the axis of embryonic development, the balance point between the upper and lower poles.

Stimulating This Meridian Line Improves the Biological Terrain in the Following Cases

In a psychological context:

to ensure vitality and a better spirit

to feel grounded

In a physical context:

to tune one's voice:

for a woman, with meridian lines 29 and 24

for a man, with meridian lines 29 and 14

to refine listening, with meridian lines 29 and 27

for hormonal balance, with meridian lines 12 and 29

for postural centering:

for a woman, with meridian lines 17 and 28

for a man, with meridian lines 17 and 21
to stimulate the gonads, with meridian line 29 and possibly:
for a woman, add meridian lines 33 and 35 to refine female expression
for a man, add meridian lines 33 and 36 to refine male expression
fragile ankles, with meridian lines 17 and 29

Meridian Line 23 of Representation

Balances the Vital Currents of the Retina

Meridian line 23 is a secondary meridian line of the Kidneys/Bladder family, which modulates the reception of all images according to the projected view (meridian 32). While the Retina is a receptor of the central nervous system, the quality of the received image depends on the projection of our eyesight. It corresponds to the point of view we have on what we see, assured by the anterior chamber of the eye. This meridian line controls the balance of visual reception, ensured by the posterior chamber of the eye: Retina and vitreous humor. This meridian line balances the exchanges on the cerebrospinal fluid level.

Stimulating This Meridian Line Improves the Biological Terrain in the Following Cases

In a psychological context:
lack of receptivity, with meridian line 09
the desire to see reality differently than it is, to live in illusions, with meridian line 31

In a physical context:
vision disturbed by fears, with meridian lines 22 and 31
to refine vision, nourish the sensor of the sight by adding meridian line 32

Meridian Line 27 of Time

Balances the Vital Currents of the Thyroid

Meridian line 27 controls the Thyroid, the "biological clock" that coordinates rhythms and time. This gland, animated by its meridian line, appears as of the seventeenth day of intrauterine life and governs the development of the child's nervous system throughout pregnancy. Any Thyroid deficiency of the mother during this period will affect the child's cerebral balance. Throughout life, this meridian line controls the basal metabolism. Associated with meridian line 13 of the Small Intestine, it controls the lipid metabolism.

This meridian line controls being in the present. It can be disrupted by a difficult move, a death, or an important shock, which can cause a temporal blockage of the individual, usually expressed by phrases such as: "my life stopped the day that . . ."

Stimulating This Meridian Line Improves the Biological Terrain in the Following Cases

In a psychological context:

- loss of temporal landmarks
- feeling of not being present during one's action, or one's life
- for adapting to the biannual time changes
- lack of stability, related to a move or relocation:
  - for a woman, with meridian line 28
  - for a man, with meridian line 21
- problems with communication, lacking listening skills, with meridian lines 09 and 29

In a physical context:

- problems with the thyroid gland:
  - for a woman, with meridian lines 35 and 37
  - for a man, with meridian lines 36 and 38
- for traveling, jet lag, with meridian line 26
- work shift adjustments
- cervical (neck) pain, with meridian line 17
- lipidic disturbances, with meridian line 13
- balance of the protein metabolism, with meridian line 18
- laryngeal problems:
  - for a woman, with meridian lines 24 and 28
  - for a man, with meridian lines 14 and 21

Meridian Line 29 of Receptivity

Balances the Vital Currents of the Veins

At the beginning of life, this meridian line supports genetic communication through the Water element, primordial fluid in which fecundation takes place.

It ensures the transmission of parental information, associated with meridian line 09. The joint action of these two meridian lines represents the similar communication between a sperm and ovum (fig. 7.4). Meridian line 29 takes part, along with meridian line 01 of the Arteries, in the balance of blood circulation in a "back and forth" exchange.

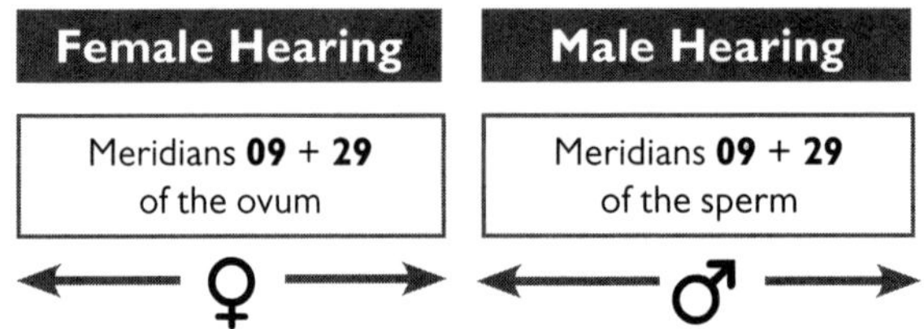

Fig. 7.4. The joint action of meridian lines 09 and 29 represents the similar communication between a sperm and ovum.

Stimulating This Meridian Line Improves the Biological Terrain in the Following Cases

In a psychological context:

communication problems, lacking listening skills, with meridian lines 09 and 27;

lacking receptivity, with meridian line 23

In a physical context:

hormonal balance, with meridian lines 12 and 29

to tune one's voice:

- for a woman, with meridian lines 29 and 24
- for a man, with meridian lines 29 and 14

balancing blood pressure, with meridian lines 01, 04, and 22

to regulate venous circulation, with meridian line 01

to stimulate the gonads, with meridian line 09 and possibly:

- for a woman, with meridian lines 33 and 35 to refine female expression
- for a man, with meridian lines 33 and 36 to refine male expression

for ankle pain, with meridian lines 09 and 17

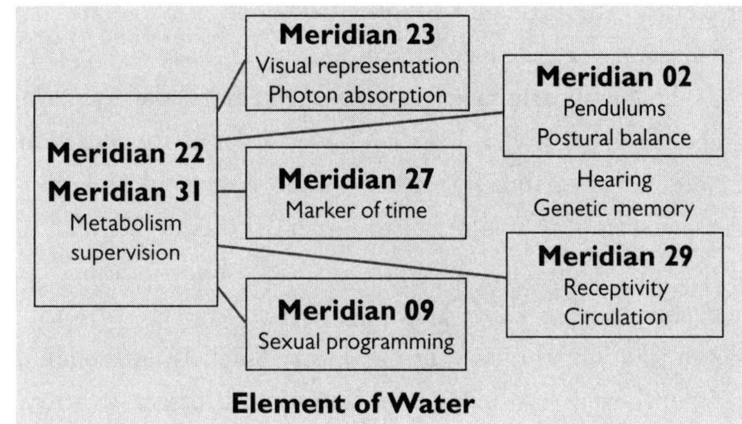

Fig. 7.5. Kidneys/ Bladder Family: communication through the element of Water

STOMACH/SPLEEN-PANCREAS FAMILY—EARTH—TASTE

The two main meridian lines of this family are 10 (Stomach) and 18 (Pancreas), combined with the secondary meridian lines 17 (Bone), 21/28 (Prostate for men/ Uterus for women), and 26 (Thalamus). Every meridian line of this family plays a core role in our psychological and behavioral dynamic.

This family guides action (10), transformation (18), and realization (21/28) in a very structured way (17) in relation to the central nervous system's core motor (26). Thus by the action of its two principal meridian lines (10 and 18) and of the secondary meridian lines, this pair governs the protein construction of tissues.

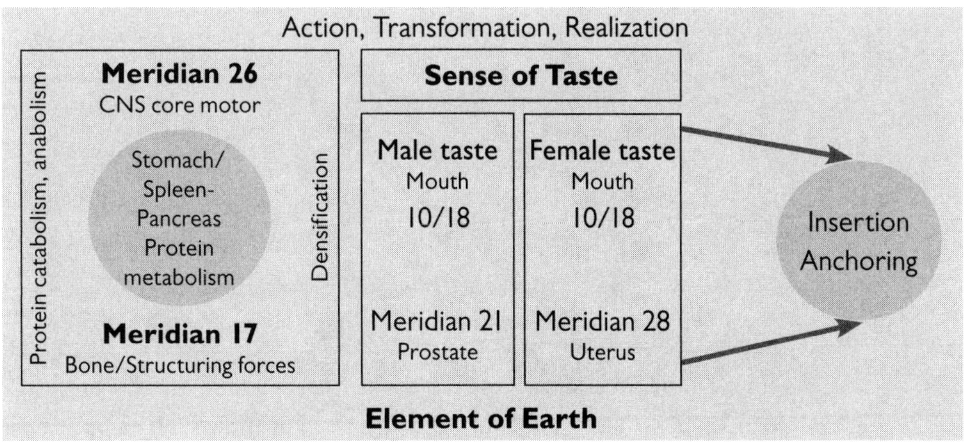

Fig. 7.6. Stomach/Spleen-Pancreas Family: meridian lines 10 and 18

It controls the anabolic/catabolic balance of protein—and structures the body by modulating the centripetal forces.

This family also manages the sense of taste: the zest for life, to manifest, act, and change—to realize oneself. This sense forms the core around which each of us builds our personality. Its activity is important at the time the seasons change; these are moments of transition between two families of meridian lines. It is particularly active during late summer, a period that Eastern tradition regards as the fifth season, the return to Earth. Indeed, after the summer—a time of plans and projects, desires that are animated by the Heart/Small Intestine family—the time is now ripe for moving into action with the Stomach/Spleen-Pancreas family.

Meridian Line 10 of Action

Balances the Vital Currents of the Stomach

Because of its pathway's destination, this meridian line acts on the balance of the Stomach, master of the action enabling us to anchor ourselves in life.

In laboratory animals, it has been observed that when all freedom of action was removed, they got ulcers, identified as "caused by constraint." In fact only an action should be undertaken that is guided by the desire of doing it, depending on the individual's capacities and genetic potential (meridian lines of the Kidneys/Bladder family).

Stimulating This Meridian Line Improves the Biological Terrain in the Following Cases

In a psychological context:

- forced action without respect for one's capacities
- loss of interest in work, idleness
- individual dominated by work
- for better coping with the end of summer and the periods the seasons change, add meridian line 18

In a physical context:

- digestive problems, gastric discomfort
- demineralization, with meridian lines 17 and 18
- acid reflux (in the pregnant woman or otherwise) with meridian line 33

This meridian line, associated with 18 (Spleen-Pancreas), is related to the sense of taste: evident in the joy of eating, being action-oriented, achieving, creating, self-realization, and manifesting life.

Meridian Line 18 of Transformation

Balances the Vital Currents of the Spleen-Pancreas

While meridian line 10 (Stomach) directs action, meridian line 18 (Spleen-Pancreas) participates in the metabolic part of transformation. It controls in particular the balance of glucids, a necessary fuel for movement of the body.

Meridian line 18 bears the name of two organs that in the Western approach apparently do not have a direct relationship. On the other hand, Eastern tradition combines the Pancreas and Spleen, thereby combining two functions essential in the transformation of tissues: solid elements (food) and liquid elements (blood).

Stimulating This Meridian Line Improves the Biological Terrain in the Following Cases

In a psychological context:

- to act freely and not only out of obligation
- taking pleasure in work
- authoritarianism, disrespectful of other people's freedom
- lack of realization in one's life, with meridian line 33
- lack of structure, lacking balance, with meridian line 17
- to better assimilate the end of the summer and the inter-seasons, combine with meridian line 10

In a physical context:

- For skeletal balance:
  - for women, with meridian lines 17 and 37
  - for men, with meridian lines 17 and 38
- any pancreatic disturbance
- demineralization, with meridian lines 10 and 17
- balance of the protein metabolism, with meridian line 27
- osteomuscular balance during growth, with meridian lines 16 and 17
- to facilitate digestion, with meridian line 11

Meridian Line 17 of Structuring

Balances the Vital Currents of the Skeletal Frame

Meridian line 17 governs the most solid element of the organism, Bone, which provides height and foundation to humans. It is involved in the balance of the osseous frame. The skeleton, the densest element of the body, is alive. Its center contains bone marrow from which are born all the blood elements.

This secondary meridian line exhibits the duality specific to the Spleen-Pancreas: the solid and liquid elements. Each bone and joint is in connection with a precise meridian line and is combined with the other surrounding meridian lines. When it is combined with the Stomach/Spleen-Pancreas couple, meridian line 17 controls the knee joint; with the Kidneys/Bladder meridian line, the ankle joint.

Stimulating This Meridian Line Improves the Biological Terrain in the Following Cases

In a psychological context:

- depressive conditions due to lack of concretization
- lack of structure, or balance, with meridian line 18

In a physical context:

- lack of flexibility, with meridian line 16
- balance of the osseous frame:
  - for women, with meridian lines 18 and 37
  - for men, with meridian lines 18 and 38
- to ensure postural centering:
  - for women, with meridian lines 09 and 28
  - for men, with meridian lines 09 and 21
- postural balance, with meridian lines 16, 33, and 34
- to accelerate the consolidation/repair of fractures
- osteoarticular flexibility:
  - for women, with meridian lines 16, 17, and 24
  - for men, with meridian lines 16, 17, and 14
- stiffness of the spinal column, with meridian lines 22 and 31
- osteomuscular balance during growth, with meridian lines 16 and 18
- demineralization, with meridian lines 10 and 18
- excessive osseous thickening, with meridian lines 22 and 31
- osseous inflammations, with meridian lines 01 and 11

Action of Meridian Line 17 on the Various Joints

cervical fragility:
- for women, with meridian lines 27
- for men, with meridian lines 27

weakness of the shoulder:
- for women, with meridian lines 05, 13, and 37
- for men, with meridian lines 05, 13, and 38

weakness of the elbow:
- for women, with meridian lines 35 and 37
- for men, with meridian lines 36 and 38

weakness of the wrist, with meridian line 04

weakness of the hip:
- for women, with meridian lines 07 and 30
- for men, with meridian lines 06 and 30

weakness of the knee:
- for women, with meridian line 28
- for men, with meridian line 21

weakness of the ankle, with meridian lines 09 and 29

Meridian Lines of Anchoring and Realization

Meridian line 21 (Prostate) in the man and 28 (Uterus) in the woman are the two meridian lines related to issues involved with setting down roots and working in a particular space. They allow us to settle down, to establish harmony with land, as well as to conceive and achieve plans. When making an intercontinental journey, it is important to control these meridian lines, in combination with meridian line 27, to fit into the new location and regulate our biorhythms.

Meridian Line 21 of Anchoring and Realization

Balances the Vital Currents of the Prostate

Meridian line 21 is a secondary meridian line that adapts male capacity for realization, governed by the Stomach/Spleen-Pancreas family.

This meridian line animates the man's taste to express life in a projective way, embodying his aspirations to raise children and assume the duties of fatherhood or to be driven to achieve success in his profession. It also controls finding the right fit with a place and setting down roots there: "settling down." This meridian line is often disrupted in people who have been uprooted from their homes and are having a hard time adjusting to a new place and time zone. It is the meridian line to be supported in case of jet lag, in combination with meridian line 27.

Stimulating This Meridian Line Improves the Biological Terrain in the Following Cases

In a psychological context:

- to find the joy in living and the desire to engender, with meridian line 33
- to live according to one's own taste
- behavioral instability (as a side effect), with meridian line 04
- for those who do not have their feet on the ground, children or adults "floating in the clouds," dreamers
- absenteeism
- difficulties of feeling comfortable with a new location, after a move or time change, with meridian line 27 (see fig. 7.7)

In a physical context:

- after dental care (any procedure in the mouth disturbs the sense of the taste), with meridian line 26
- balance of the male genital sphere, with meridian line 06
- to support postural balance, with meridian lines 09 and 17
- prostatic disorders, in conjunction with common medication
- knee problems for a man, with meridian line 17
- laryngeal demonstration for a man, with the meridian lines 27 and 14

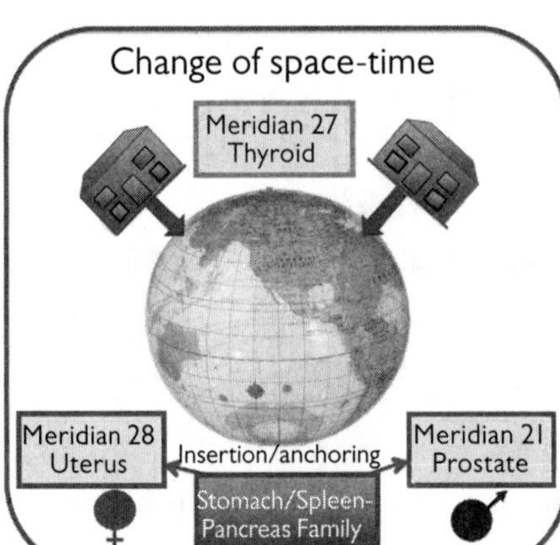

Fig. 7.7. Moving to a new home

Meridian Line 28 of Anchoring and Realization

Balances the Vital Currents of the Uterus

Meridian line 28 (Uterus) is a secondary meridian line that outlines female capacity for realization and achievement, governed by the Stomach/Spleen-Pancreas family. In women it shapes the zest for life whether it is the desire to become a mother or find self-fulfillment in work. It also regulates finding the right fit with a living space and setting down roots: settling down. Women are affected by disruptions of this meridian line. In addition to dealing with jet lag, women can support this meridian line for help in dealing with low fertility, in combination with meridian line 24 (Breasts).

Stimulating This Meridian Line Improves the Biological Terrain in the Following Cases

In a psychological context:

- difficulty living to one's own taste, and fear of not pleasing someone else
- to find the autonomy in a concrete action
  - for those who do not have their "feet on the ground," children or adults with "head in the clouds," dreamers
- lack of joy in expressing life, including giving birth
- trouble coping with being a mother, with meridian lines 24 and 33

In a physical context:

- after dental care (any procedure in the mouth disturbs the sense of taste), with meridian line 26
- difficulty in adjusting to a new location (sometimes caused by depression after a move, or while traveling), for better finding oneself, with meridian line 27 (fig. 7.7)
- emotional instability, with meridian line 04
- to ensure postural centering, with meridian lines 09 and 17
- disorders of the uterus, menstrual contractions
- balance of the female genital sphere, with meridian line 07
- contractions at the beginning of gestation, nausea, dislike of pregnancy (reduced desire to give birth), with meridian lines 24 and 33
- difficulty conceiving, with meridian line 24 and 33
- laryngeal problems for a woman, with meridian lines 24 and 27
- knee problems for a woman, with meridian line 17

The Uterus is a place of life, of creation; it expresses the desire to exist and allows implantation and construction of life. Implantation evokes fitting in into a place and the ability to set down roots there.

Meridian Line 26 of Motor Conduction

Balances the Vital Currents of the Cerebral Motor System/Gray Matter

The cerebral motor system is the starting point for action and movement. Meridian line 26 controls the cerebral motor system, in relation to the sense of taste (meridian lines 21 for a man or 28 for a woman).

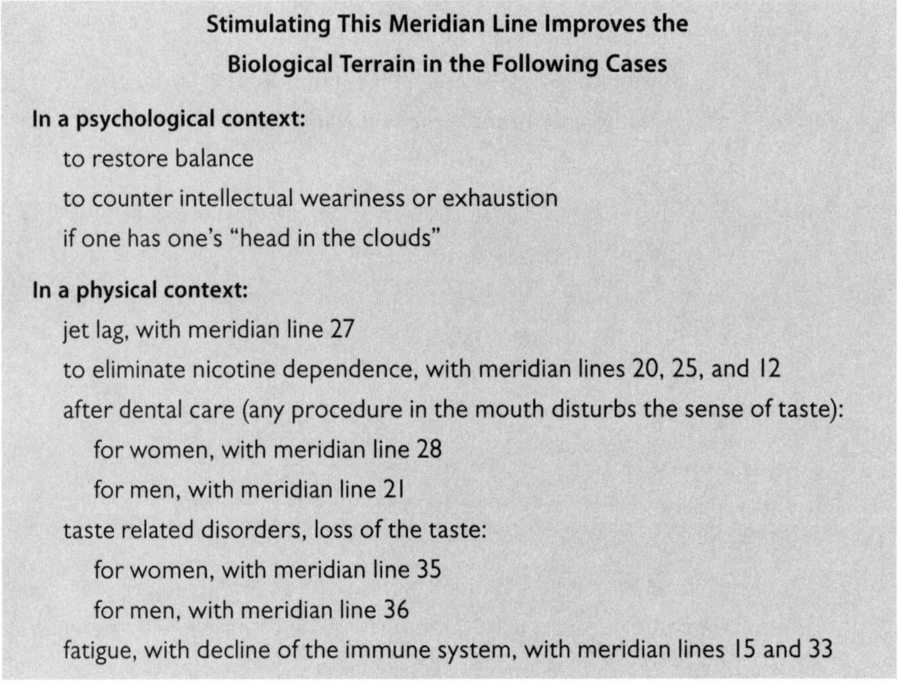

Stimulating This Meridian Line Improves the Biological Terrain in the Following Cases

In a psychological context:

- to restore balance
- to counter intellectual weariness or exhaustion
- if one has one's "head in the clouds"

In a physical context:

- jet lag, with meridian line 27
- to eliminate nicotine dependence, with meridian lines 20, 25, and 12
- after dental care (any procedure in the mouth disturbs the sense of taste):
  - for women, with meridian line 28
  - for men, with meridian line 21
- taste related disorders, loss of the taste:
  - for women, with meridian line 35
  - for men, with meridian line 36
- fatigue, with decline of the immune system, with meridian lines 15 and 33

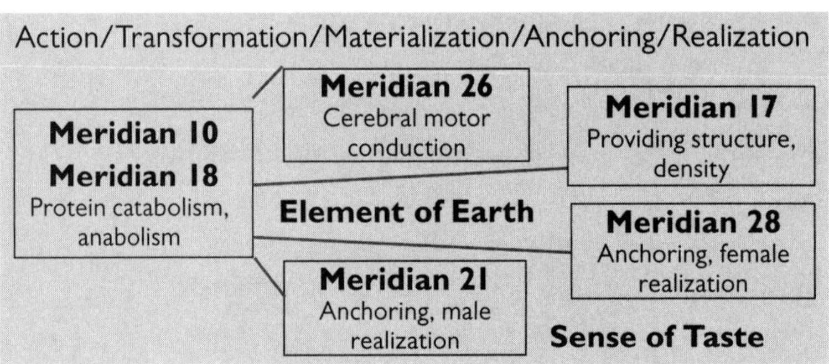

Fig. 7.8. Stomach/Spleen-Pancreas Family

LIVER/GALLBLADDER FAMILY—BOUNDARY/ETHER—TOUCH

This pair of meridian lines, 11 (Liver) and 30 (Gall Bladder), represents the blood metabolic pole of the organism, governing the action of the Kidneys/Bladder and Stomach/Spleen-Pancreas pairs. Its action is complementary to that of the neural cerebral pole, directed by the main meridian lines, Master of the Heart and Triple Warmer, which hold its nourishing impulse.

Meridian Line 11 of Metabolic Activation

Balances the Vital Currents of the Liver

Meridian Line 11 governing metabolic activation is complementary with meridians lines 35/36 of neural activation. This meridian line 11 is the quintessential nourishing meridian line since it controls the development of all the nutritional elements necessary to cells (A.T.P.), provided by the Liver. It is an important line to regulate when feeling a lack of energy. Combined with the Gall Bladder meridian, the Liver meridian represents the metabolic pole. The highest demands are placed on it during the spring season.

Stimulating This Meridian Line Improves the Biological Terrain in the Following Cases

In a psychological context:

- choleric temperament or, to the contrary, depressive tendencies
- mental and intellectual overwork, depression, with meridian lines 08 and 12
- to better cope with spring:
  - for women, with meridian lines 30, 35, and 37
  - for men, with meridian lines 30, 36, and 38

In a physical context:

- chronic exhaustion, overwork, with meridian line 30
- any hepatic demonstration: it brings an effective help in addition to common medication
- detoxification capacities for the organism, with meridian line 30
- assistance with digestion, with meridian line 18
- any inflammation problems, with meridian line 01

osseous inflammations, with meridian lines 01 and 17
muscular coordination:
for women, with meridian lines 16, 30, 35, and 37
for men, with meridian lines 16, 30, 36, and 38
any cutaneous manifestation, with meridian lines 19 and 30, to help with current medication
all capillary problems, with meridian line 19
seborrheic dermatitis affecting the scalp, with meridian lines 03, 19, and 30
skin with acne-prone tendencies, with meridian lines 01 and 19

Meridian Line 30 of Metabolic Regulation

Balances the Vital Currents of the Gall Bladder

Meridian line 30 (Gall Bladder) regulates the flow of metabolic energy and the activity of meridian line 11. It encourages biliary evacuation, and supports the general drainage of the organism. This line should always be given stimulation when dealing with metabolic plethora and blood overloads. Coupled with meridian lines 11 and 01, it controls cutaneous problems and inflammatory processes. It is more particularly active during the season of spring.

Stimulating This Meridian Line Improves the Biological Terrain in the Following Cases

In a psychological context:
aggressive characters, suffering from "mood swings"
people full of rancor, bitterness
choleric temperaments, with meridian line 11
to better cope with spring:
for women, with meridian lines 11, 35, and 37
for men, with meridian lines 11, 36, and 38

In a physical context:
any disturbance of the Gall Bladder, with some type of "biliary idleness," "bilious attack"
physical exhaustion, overwork, with meridian line 11
any phenomenon of excess blood in the circulatory system:
for women, with meridian line 37
for men, with meridian line 38

purgative and detoxification action of the organism, with meridian line 11
after general anesthesia, with meridian lines 08 and 12
muscular coordination:
  for women, with meridian lines 16, 11, 35, and 37
  for men, with meridian lines 16, 11, 36, and 38
filtration of waste:
  for women, with meridian lines 01 and 37
  for men, with meridian lines 01 and 38
any cutaneous manifestation, often in conjunction with meridian lines 11 and 19, to assist common medication
all capillary problems, with meridian line 19
seborrheic dermatitis (dandruff) of the scalp, with meridian lines 11, 19, and 03
weaknesses of the hips:
  for women, with meridian lines 07 and 17
  for men, with meridian lines 06 and 17
weakness of the shoulders:
  for women, with meridian lines 05, 13, 17, and 37
  for men, with meridian lines 05, 13, 17, and 38

Note: The activity of the Liver/Gall Bladder family is complementary to that of the Master of Heart/Triple Warmer family. These two families jointly govern the dynamics of the two principal poles of the organism—metabolic and cerebral.

8
The Rhythmic Meridians of the Upper Body

WHILE THE MERIDIAN LINES of the lower body provide a sure supply of the essential energy to build life, the rhythmic meridian lines of the upper body adjust them and express all their subtleties. The rhythmic families—Lungs/Colon, Heart/Small Intestine, and Master of the Heart/Triple Warmer—also preside over individual cognitive maturation.

The Lungs/Colon family, in connection with the Air element, governs the sense of smell. It permits an integration of one's gender and combines it with the sexual reality of the body with the secondary sexual organs. These meridian lines are very active during puberty to ensure the regulation of the hormonal system, which allows the transformation of the young girl and the young boy with the appearance of the main organs from this phase (Breasts and Adam's Apple/Larynx).

Meanwhile the Heart/Small Intestine family, related to the Fire element, gives access to individual consciousness, to project oneself in life guided by the individual's desire to exist.

A third pair of meridian lines, Master of the Heart/Triple Warmer, govern the cerebral pole, complementary to the blood metabolic pole, whose synergy is essential to ensure the bipolar balance of the organism.

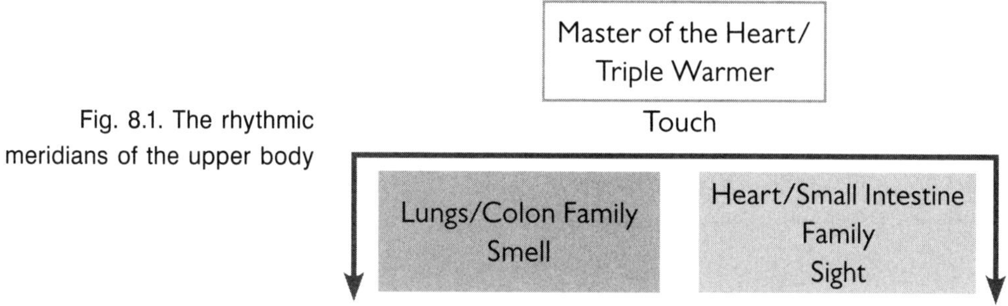

Fig. 8.1. The rhythmic meridians of the upper body

LUNGS/COLON FAMILY—AIR—SMELL

The meridians of this family are related to the element of Air, and govern the sense of smell and sexual expression. This family has a greater sensitivity in autumn. This family includes many secondary meridian lines for both men and women. Two particular meridian lines control the sexual expression of the upper body: meridian line 24 (Breasts) for women and meridian line 14 (Adam's Apple/Larynx) for men.

This family has a connection to the rhinencephalic hormonal system, which manages sexual instinctive impulses normally modulated by the cerebral cortex—the pole of consciousness in human beings. It receives, via meridian line 15, governing self-expression, the distillate of physical metabolic manifestations ensured by the lymphatic system.

Inhalation, conducted by meridians 20 of breath and 25 of inspiration, enables the individual through his rhinencephalic and meridian line 12 of instinct to perceive

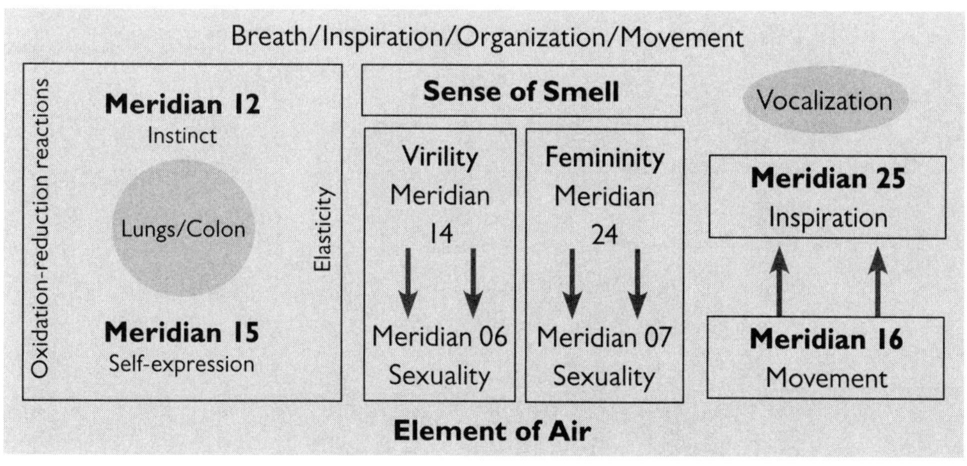

Fig. 8.2. Lungs/Colon Family: meridian lines 20 and 05, communication through the element Air

fragrance and identify it. This makes it possible for the sense of smell to direct metabolic action, "to clue the individual in" according to her female or his male sensitivity. Each individual's actions are organized by the other meridian lines of this family: 05 and 06 for men and 05 and 07 for women. We can summarize the expression of this couple with this hierarchical dynamics: inhalation (meridian line 20) governs individual organization (meridian line 05).

Meridian Line 20 of Breath

Balances the Vital Currents of the Lungs

Meridian line 20 is a fundamental circuit that manifests in the baby's first cry upon coming into this world. Breathing is a semi-voluntary act, modulated by each person's relational difficulties, and their rigid or expansive attitude toward life. It is the meridian line of movement, flexibility, and openness to the world.

Stimulating This Meridian Line Improves the Biological Terrain in the Following Cases

In a psychological context:

- to overcome excessive idealism, perfectionism, conformism, dogmatic attitudes
- to find more hope in life, with meridian line 05
- lack of inspiration, with meridian lines 12 and 25
- to catch one's breath for everyday activities, with meridian line 16
- to better acclimate to the season of autumn, with meridian line 05

In a physical context:

- transitory disorders, with meridian lines 05, 16, and 33
- excessive perfectionism, obsessive tendencies, which translates into lack of flexibility:
  - for women, with meridian lines 07 and 05
  - for men, with meridian lines 06 and 05
- any skin manifestation, often in conjunction with meridian lines 11 and 30, to assist common medication
- lack of elasticity in skin, with meridian line 20
- respiratory problems, with meridian lines 15 and 25
- to overcome nicotine or tobacco dependence, with meridian lines 25, 12, and 26

This meridian line controls breathing, offering flexibility and self-confidence. It encourages individual expression and modulates male or female sexual sensibility. It is more particularly sensitive during the season of autumn.

Meridian Line 05 of Organization

Balances the Vital Currents of the Colon

While meridian line 20 manages breathing, meridian line 05 governs individual organization. When the organization gains the upper hand over breathing, various disorders (related to this reversal of information between the meridian line of the Lung and that of the Colon) can appear. The individual can lose his breath, his inspiration, and become disorganized, He can behave in a constrained, rigid fashion when severed from his own breathing (inspiration).

Meridian line 05 also plays a big role in sexual expression. Its dynamics are formed during the evolutionary stages of early childhood. Depending on the individual's lifestyle, in particular during the anal stage, interference can happen on the balance of this meridian line. Any event that obstructs the faculty of individual organization can induce a psychological contraction, often the source of dry bowel movements and constipation, and a kind of mental inflexibility.

Stimulating This Meridian Line Improves the Biological Terrain in the Following Cases

In a psychological context:

- difficulties organizing
- to feel more hopeful in life, with meridian line 05
- excessive perfectionism, obsessive tendency, which translates to a lack of flexibility:
  - for women, with meridian lines 07 and 20
  - for men, with meridian lines 06 and 20
- for better acclimating to the season of autumn, with meridian line 20

In a physical context:

- occasional constipation, with meridian line 16
- disorders affecting the elimination of wastes, with meridian lines 16, 20, and 33
- digestive, abdominal discomfort, with meridian line 16

shoulder pain:
- for women, with meridian lines 17, 13, and 37
- for men, with meridian lines 17, 13, and 38

Meridian Line 12 of Instinct

Balances the Vital Currents of the Hypothalamus

Meridian line 12 plays a fundamental role in the hormonal fluctuations. It is in relation to the rhinencephalon, the oldest part of the brain, which collects the olfactory impulses interfering with hormonal secretions. This meridian line is particularly sensitive to stress and physical and intellectual overwork.

Stimulating This Meridian Line Improves the Biological Terrain in the Following Cases

In a psychological context:

- mental and intellectual overwork, depressive tendencies, with meridian lines 08 and 11
- loss of one's female or male sensitivity:
  - for women, with meridian line 24
  - for men, with meridian line 14

In a physical context:

- to overcome nicotine dependence, with meridian lines 20, 25, and 26
- hormonal balance, with meridian lines 09 and 29
- to stimulate general defenses, with meridian lines 15 and 25
- to prepare for taking school examinations, with meridian line 08
- after surgical operation under general anesthesia, with meridian lines 08 and 30
- reduction in the sense of smell:
  - for women, with meridian lines 07 and 25
  - for men, with meridian lines 06 and 25
- nasal discharge:
  - for women, with meridian lines 25 and 37
  - for men, with meridian lines 25 and 38
- For athletes, for optimal muscular dynamics and fast recovery, with meridian lines 02, 08, and 16

Meridian Line 15 of Self-Expression

Balances the Vital Currents of the Lymphatic System

Meridian line 15 supports the immune system. It guarantees the integrity of the self and protects the body from foreign elements.

While meridian line 01 (Gift) transmits the necessary information for cellular life, meridian line 29 (Receptivity) ensures the return, and meridian line 15 (Self-expression) transports the information "distilled" by the cell. The lymph is indeed a byproduct of cellular work. It expresses each individual's profound reality, his uniqueness and singular odor. It is what enables us, along with the sense of smell, to be able to distinguish one person from another. This sense is exaggerated in most animals (in relation to the rhinencephalon), whereas in humans the system of recognition and choice is our more developed sense of sight (in connection with the cerebral cortex).

Stimulating This Meridian Line Improves the Biological Terrain in the Following Cases

In a psychological context:

intolerant behavior

In a physical context:

respiratory problems, with meridian lines 20 and 25
to reinforce general defenses, with meridian lines 12 and 25
balance of vaginal flora, with meridian line 07
fatigue, with lowered immunity, with meridian lines 26 and 33

Meridian Line 16 of Movement

Balances the Vital Currents of the Muscles

It is the meridian line of movement, supplied by the breath. When combined with the five families of meridian lines, it expresses various muscular qualities: force, tonicity, elasticity, impulse, and coordination.

With the Lungs/Colon family, it ensures muscular flexibility. With the Stomach/Spleen-Pancreas family it ensures strength; with the Kidneys/Bladder family, tonicity. With the Heart/Small Intestine couple, it encourages muscular impulse. Finally, with the Master of the Heart/Triple Warmer and Liver/Gall Bladder couples it coordinates and feeds movement.

Stimulating This Meridian Line Improves the Biological Terrain in the Following Cases

In a psychological context:

for tense people, contracted musculature, lacking flexibility
lack of expansiveness

In a physical context:

neuro-muscular stiffness, muscular aches, spasms (smooth fibers and striated fibers)
occasional constipation, with meridian line 05
eliminatory disorders, with meridian lines 05, 20, and 33
osteo-muscular balance during growth, with meridian lines 17 and 18
to take a "breather" between everyday activities, with meridian line 20
for athletes, before and after sports, it allows an optimal muscular function and a fast recovery, with meridian lines 02, 08, and 12

On the osteomuscular level it ensures:

the balance of the osteomuscular frame, with meridian lines 17 and 18
osteoarticular flexibility:
- for women, with meridian lines 17 and 24
- for men, with meridian lines 17 and 14

postural balance, with meridian lines 17, 33, and 34
muscular flexibility, with meridian lines 05 and 20
muscle tone, with meridian lines 22 and 31
muscular impulse, with meridian lines 04 and 13
muscle strength, with meridian lines 10 and 18
muscular coordination:
- for women, with meridian lines 35, 37, 11, and 30
- for men, with meridian lines 36, 38, 11, and 30

This meridian line controls the balance of the muscular system, anatomically located in a median position between the skin and the bone. The precise spatial orientation for these three sections of the body, with respect to the body diagram, is fundamental for ensuring our ability to perform to the best of our abilities. A spatial confusion between skin, muscles, and bone has been observed in some people, causing a "threading error" of the corresponding meridian lines, creating spasms and muscle contractions. The information conveyed by meridian lines 19, 16, and 17 is therefore delivered in a chaotic manner causing short circuits, which are responsible for various disorders. Although the cause for this spatial confusion remains unknown, it has proven to be a smart idea to stimulate these meridian lines in order to ensure their harmonious interaction, as this is the basis for good postural balance.

Meridian Line 25 of Inspiration

Balances the Vital Currents of the Sinus

Meridian line 25 is connected with air communication and, in synergy with meridian line 12 (Hypothalamus), also has an action on smell. It nourishes the vital currents of the Sinuses and the rhinopharynx. A balanced Sinus system is the reflection of good respiratory dynamics, flavored by one's sensitivity, female or male (fig. 8.3).

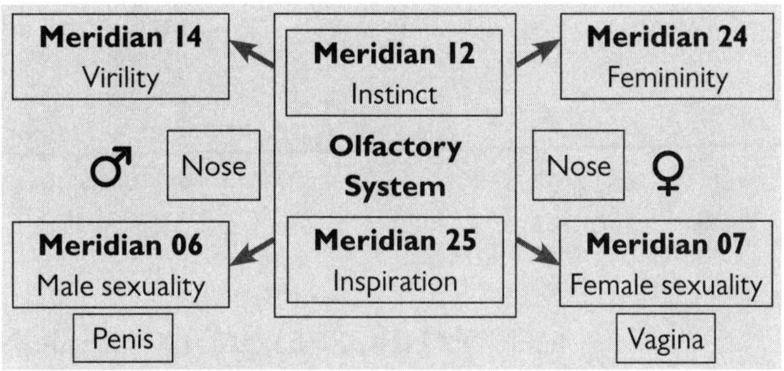

Fig. 8.3. The sense of smell

Stimulating This Meridian Line Improves the Biological Terrain in the Following Cases

In a psychological context:

poor expression of what one feels, not trusting one's own feelings, with meridian lines 12 and 20

In a physical context:

to overcome nicotine dependence, with meridian lines 20, 12, and 26

any disturbance of the sinuses

to stimulate the overall defense system, with meridian lines 12 and 15

allergies, often due to disturbances in the relations with the outside world

the first signs of flu-like symptoms, e.g., sneezes

nasal discharge:
- for women, with meridian lines 12 and 37
- for men, with meridian lines 12 and 38

respiratory disorders, with meridian lines 15 and 20

olfactory weakness:
- for women, with meridian lines 07 and 12
- for men, with meridian lines 06 and 12

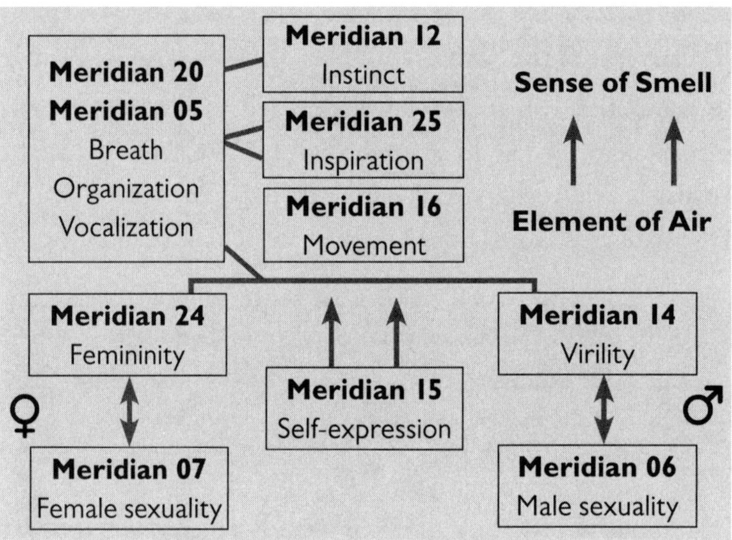

Fig. 8.4 Lungs/Colon Family: communication through the element Air

MERIDIANS OF SEXUAL EXPRESSION

Meridian Line 06 of Male Sexuality

Balances the Vital Currents of the Penis

This meridian line has an action on the dynamic of the sexual pole. When it is well-balanced, it ensures the man all his male prowess and allows him to express his virility. It interacts with meridian lines 24 and 05.

Stimulating This Meridian Line Improves the Biological Terrain in the Following Cases

In a psychological context:

difficulties in expressing ones virility, with meridian lines 14 and 36

lacking male expression, with meridian lines 36 and 38

In a physical context:

any erectile performance, as a complement to standard medications, with meridian lines 14 and 36

hip pain for a man, with meridian lines 17 and 30

reduction in the sense of smell for a man, with meridian lines 12 and 25

to balance the male genital sphere, with meridian line 21

Meridian Line 07 of the Vagina

Balances the Vital Currents of the Vagina

The dynamics of this meridian line ensure a radiant sexual life. Its regulating action on the sexual pole enables the woman to open up and express all her femininity. It is connected with meridian lines 24 and 05, with which it interacts quite closely.

Stimulating This Meridian Line Improves the Biological Terrain in the Following Cases

In a psychological context:

sexual denial, with meridian lines 35 and 37

In a physical context:

for all vaginal performance, as a supplement to standard medication

balance of the female genital sphere, with meridian line 28

to refine the sense of smell for women, with meridian lines 12 and 25

hot flashes, with meridian lines 24 and 37

balance of vaginal flora, with meridian line 15

to support a radiant sexual life, with the meridian line 24

hip pain for a woman, with meridian lines 17 and 30

Meridian Line 14 of Virility

Balances the Vital Currents of the Adam's Apple

This is the meridian line that expresses virility. With puberty, the voice of the young boy changes, it breaks and becomes gradually deeper. The larynx, more prominent, causes the Adam's Apple to stand out.

Each Sector of the Sexual Pole Is Animated by One of the Five Elements

The meridians of the Uterus and Prostate are secondary currents of the Stomach/Spleen-Pancreas family (Earth element).

The meridians of the Gonads (ovaries and testicles) form part of the Kidneys/Bladder family (Water element).

The meridians of the Vagina and Penis are connected to the Lungs/Colon family (Air element).

The meridians of the Cervix for women and the Glans for men are related to the Heart/Small Intestine family (Fire element).

The meridians of the Vulva for women and the Scrotum for men are related to the two families of Liver/Gall Bladder and Master of the Heart/Triple Warmer (Boundary element).

Stimulating This Meridian Line Improves the Biological Terrain in the Following Cases

In a psychological context:

expression of virility, with meridian lines 06 and 38.

In a physical context:

any erectile performance, as a supplement to standard medication, with meridian lines 06 and 36

to tune one's voice, with meridian lines 29 and 09

osteo-articular flexibility, with meridian lines 16 and 17

laryngeal demonstration for a man, with meridian lines 27 and 21

Meridian Line 24 of Femininity

Balances the Vital Currents of the Breasts

Meridian line 24 supports the expression of femininity. Its disordered state can induce a sense of profound discomfort for women, which can be the source for other disorders, both psychological and physical.

Stimulating This Meridian Line Improves the Biological Terrain in the Following Cases

In a psychological context:

expression of femininity, with meridian lines 07 and 37

In a physical context:

to tune the voice, with meridian lines 29 and 09
laryngeal demonstration for a woman, with meridian lines 27 and 28
morning sickness, with meridian lines 28 and 33
harmony with maternity, with meridian lines 28 and 33
mammary disorders, as an additional therapy
hot flashes, with meridian lines 07 and 37
osteo-articular flexibility, with meridian lines 16 and 17
contractions at the beginning of gestation, with meridian lines 28 and 33
difficulties in getting pregnant, with meridian line 28 and 33

HEART/SMALL INTESTINE FAMILY—FIRE—SIGHT

The two chiefs of this family are the meridian lines 04 (Rhythm) and 13 (Choice) to which are attached three secondary meridian lines: 01 (Gift), 08 (Cognitive Integration), and 32 (View/Vision). This family, along with its relationship to the neocerebellum, characterizes the projective system of humans, which gives access to consciousness. It has a greater sensitivity in the summer.

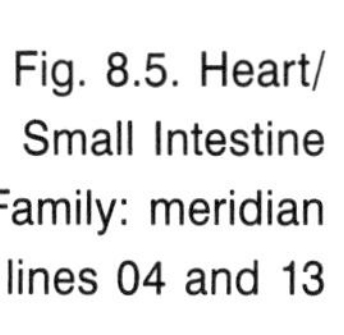
Fig. 8.5. Heart/ Small Intestine Family: meridian lines 04 and 13

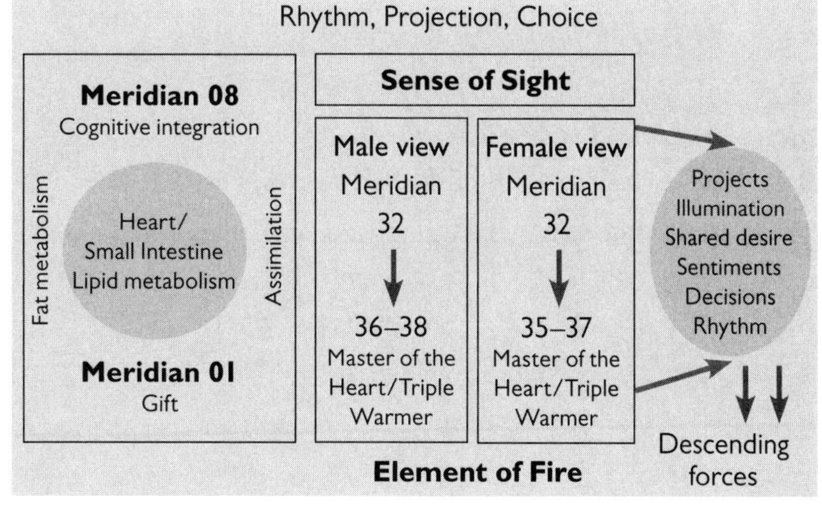

Meridian Line 04 of Projective Rhythm

Balances the Vital Currents of the Heart

Just like the Heart, which pulsates blood through the entire body, this is a meridian line that impels a projective rhythm to the entire organism. It takes part in resource sharing, in interaction with meridian lines 01 and 29.

Stimulating This Meridian Line Improves the Biological Terrain in the Following Cases

In a psychological context:

- lack of desire, unable to make plans, with meridian line 32 and 08
- lack of "get-up-and-go," with meridian line 01
- difficulties in managing one's feelings, too emotional/no objectivity
- tendency to feel guilty, to feel disliked
- difficulties in sharing, with meridian line 01
- tendency to forget the self to please others
- emotional instability:
  - for women, with meridian line 28
  - for men, with meridian line 21
- fear of not being liked, with meridian line 22
- for better acclimating to the summer season, with meridian line 13

In a physical context:

- any cardiac manifestation
- arterial circulation, with meridian line 01
- regulating blood pressure, with meridian lines 01, 22, and 29

Meridian Line 13 of Choice

Balances the Vital Currents of the Small Intestine

This meridian line regulates food/nutrition assimilation and plays a big role at the immune level (lymphocytes). At the mental level, it ensures the capacity to choose and decide. It has a greater sensitivity in summer.

Stimulating This Meridian Line Improves the Biological Terrain in the Following Cases

In a psychological context:

difficulties making decisions

difficulties in living and expressing personal choices

for better assimilating the summer season, with meridian line 04

In a physical context:

obesity with disturbance of affectivity and emotional sensitivity

lipidic disorders, with meridian line 27

shoulder pains:

- for women, with meridian lines 05, 17, and 37
- for men, with meridian lines 05, 17, and 38

Meridian Line 01 of the Gift

Balances the Vital Currents of the Arteries

This secondary meridian line supports the rhythmic impulse of meridian line 04, regulating the projection of blood into the bloodstream.

Stimulating This Meridian Line Improves the Biological Terrain in the Following Cases

In a psychological context:

lack of energy, with meridian line 04

lack of communication, with meridian line 29

difficulty sharing, with meridian line 04

In a physical context:

filtration of waste:

- for women, with meridian lines 30 and 37
- for men, with meridian lines 30 and 38

any inflammatory processes, with meridian line 11

bone inflammations, with meridian lines 11 and 17

blood pressure regulation, with meridian lines 04, 22, and 29

skin with acne tendencies, with meridian lines 11 and 19

This meridian line activates the entire arterial system:

- arterial circulation, with meridian line 04
- venous circulation, with meridian line 29

Note: Certain arterial imbalances can be related to the dysfunction of meridian line 29 (Kidneys/Bladder family). A confusion of information between the Kidneys/Bladder and Heart/Small Intestine families can involve circulatory disorders, of which one consequence can be an "informational disruption" at the thoracic level.

Meridian Line 08 of Cognitive Integration

Balances the Vital Currents of the Cerebral Cortex

This is a secondary meridian line of the Heart/Small Intestine family that made it possible for the neocerebellum to develop in human beings. Providing support to this meridian line reinforces the Cerebral Cortex and revitalizes its projective dynamics. Meridian line 08 controls the cerebral pole and offers it all the power necessary for its conduction role. It acts as a neurological regulator. This meridian line is more sensitive in the summer.

Stimulating This Meridian Line Improves the Biological Terrain in the Following Cases

general stability, with meridian line 11
inability to make plans, with meridian line 04 and 32
preparation for school examinations, with meridian line 12
after general anesthesia, with meridian lines 12 and 30
overwork, severe fatigue, with meridian lines 11 and 12
offers athletes optimal muscular dynamics and fast recovery, with meridian lines 02, 12, and 16

Meridian Line 32 of Vision

Balances the Vital Currents of Sight

This meridian line ensures the projection of sight and modulates the luminous information it receives. It is in connection with the epiphysis, which receives the information of the retina to harmonize the body's biorhythms. Meridian line 32 controls the components of the anterior chamber of the eye: cornea, aqueous humor, crystalline, iris.

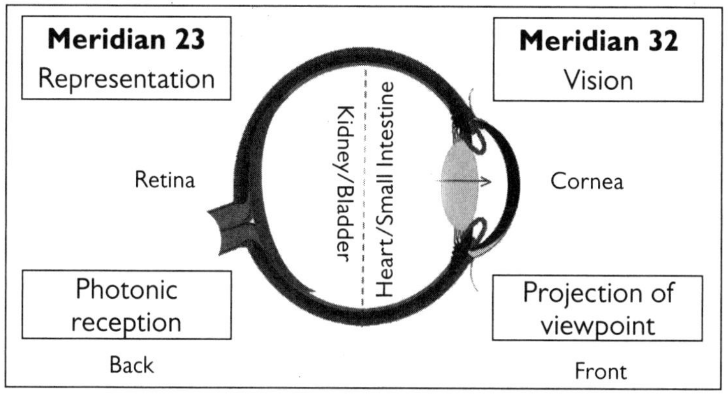

Fig. 8.6. Sense of sight

Stimulating This Meridian Line Improves the Biological Terrain in the Following Cases

lack of projection, with meridian lines 04 and 08
in any disturbance of the anterior chamber of the eye
overly sensitive to light
to nourish the sensory organ of sight, with meridian line 23

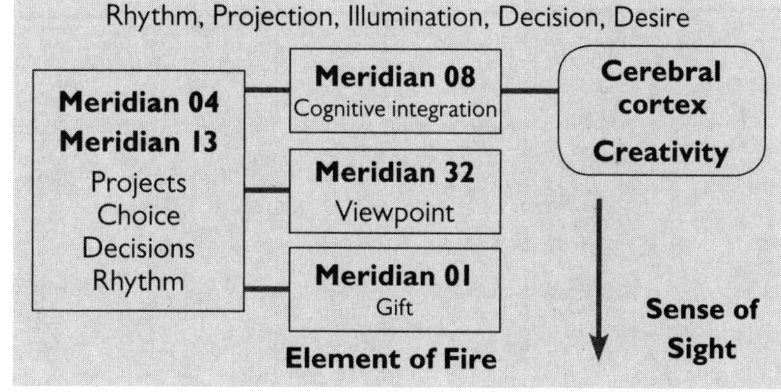

Fig. 8.7. Heart/Small Intestine Family

MERIDIAN LINES OF THE SETTING: THE CONCEPT OF COHERENCE

The meridian lines of the Master of the Heart (lines 35/36) and Triple Warmer (lines 37/38) pair coordinate the circulation of all the meridian lines and modulate the metabolic action of the Liver/Gall Bladder family. They ensure each individual characteristic form. Their primary role is to control and contain the metabolic impulse, as guards of the body's boundaries.

Although Eastern tradition integrates these meridian lines into the Heart/Small Intestine family, experiments led by Nutripuncture define this pair as being the neural "boundary" of the organism, conveying a sexual imprint. To differentiate individuals according to gender, they are: meridian lines 35/37 for a woman, and meridian lines 36/38 for a man.

We have attached two particular meridian lines to this family that govern the boundaries of the body, represented by the skin and the hair.

Meridian Line 35 of Feminine Nerve Activation

Balances the Vital Currents of the Master of the Heart for Women

Meridian line 35 for women is associated with no organ in particular, but it provides a function complementary to that of meridian line 37: regulation of the sympathetic and parasympathetic nervous system. It stimulates the conduction of all organs in conjunction with the other cerebral meridians and acts on the sexual expression. This meridian line, always in synergy with meridian line 37, contains and limits the metabolic impulse of the Liver/Gall Bladder family.

Stimulating This Meridian Line Improves the Biological Terrain in the Following Cases

In a psychological context:

apathetic temperament, with meridian line 37
lack of female expression, with meridian line 37
to support neural balance, with meridian line 37
when one feels surrounded by the wrong crowd, with meridian line 19 and 37
for better assimilation of the spring season, with meridian lines 11, 30, and 37

In a physical context:

in certain allergic disorders with loss of female polarity
to help control the autonomic nervous system
in addition to common medication for cerebral congestive disorders, with meridian line 37
loss of sensitivity, with meridian lines 02 and 37
disorders affecting the sense of taste, loss of taste, in conjunction with meridian line 26
problems with the thyroid gland, with meridian lines 27 and 37

to stimulate the gonads (ovaries), with meridian lines 09, 29, and 33
muscular coordination, with meridian lines 16, 37, 11, and 30
fragility of the elbow, with meridian lines 17 and 37

Meridian Line 36 of Male Nerve Activation

Balances the Vital Currents of the Master of the Heart for Men

Meridian line 36 in the man is associated with no organ in particular. It provides one primary function, complementary to that of meridian line 38: regulation of the sympathetic and parasympathetic nervous systems. It stimulates the conduction of all organs in conjunction with the other cerebral meridians and acts on the sexual expression. In the event of neuro-autonomic hypo-excitability, even apathy, this line stimulates nerve activity. This meridian line, always in synergy with meridian line 38, contains and limits the metabolic impulse of the Liver/Gall Bladder family.

Stimulating This Meridian Line Improves the Biological Terrain in the Following Cases

In a psychological context:

apathetic temperament, with meridian line 38
lacking male expression, with meridian line 38
to support nervous system balance, with meridian line 38
when one feels surrounded by the wrong crowd, with meridian line 19 and 38
for better assimilation of the spring season, with meridian lines 11, 30, and 38

In a physical context:

in certain allergic disorders where there is loss of male polarity
in addition to common medication for cerebral congestive disorders, with meridian line 38
any erectile dysfunction, in complement to common medication, with meridian lines 06 and 14
muscular coordination, with meridian lines 16, 38, 11, and 30
loss of sensitivity, with meridian lines 02 and 38
thyroid gland problems, with meridian lines 27 and 38
to stimulate the gonads, with meridian lines 09, 29, and 33
disorders of the sense of taste, loss of taste, in conjunction with meridian line 26
fragility of the elbow, in the man, with meridian lines 17 and 38

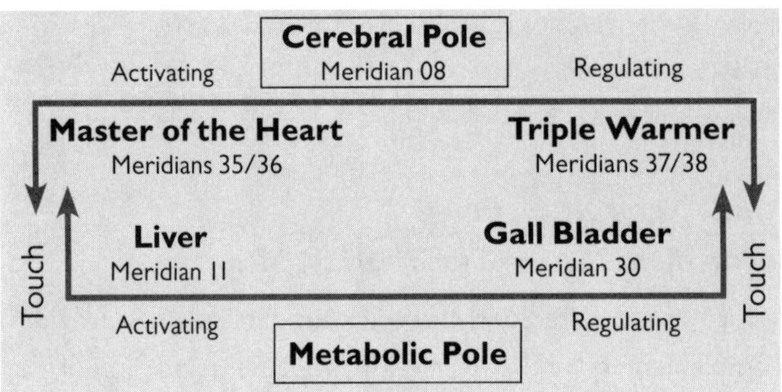

Fig. 8.8. The bipolar dynamic of the body and the meridians involved in the sense of touch

Meridian Line 37 of Female Nerve Regulation

Balances the Vital Currents of the Triple Warmer for Women

This meridian line, in women, is not connected to any organ in particular. However, its primary function is to regulate the entire body/organism. In synergy with meridian line 35 it controls the parasympathetic and sympathetic nervous systems. It brings heat and life to the neurosensory balance. It controls excesses when there is a vegetative-nervous hyper-excitability.

This meridian line, always in synergy with the meridian line 35, limits and contains the metabolic impulse of the Liver/Gall Bladder family.

Stimulating This Meridian Line Improves the Biological Terrain in the Following Cases

In a psychological context:

apathetic temperament, with meridian line 35
lacking female expression, with meridian lines 35 and 07
to control neural balance, with meridian line 35
when one feels surrounded by the wrong crowd, with meridian lines 19 and 35
for better acclimating to the spring season, with meridian lines 11, 30, and 35

In a physical context:

loss of sensitivity, with meridian lines 02 and 35
can be added to common medication for cerebral congestive disorders, with meridian line 37
flexibility of the skin, with meridian line 19
filtration of waste, with meridian lines 30 and 01
hot flashes, with meridian lines 24 and 07

thyroid gland problems, with meridian lines 35 and 27
fragility of the elbow in women, with meridian lines 17 and 35
nasal discharge, with meridian lines 12 and 25
fragility of the shoulders in women, with meridian lines 05, 17, and 13
urinary problems, with meridian lines 22, 31, and 33
muscular coordination, with meridian lines 16, 35, 11, and 30
any phenomenon of plethora, with meridian line 30
skeletal balance, with meridian lines 18 and 17

Meridian Line 38 of Male Nerve Regulation

Balances the Vital Currents of the Triple Warmer for Men

This meridian line in men is not connected to any organ in particular. It primarily provides one function: regulation of the entire organism. In synergy with meridian line 37, it controls the parasympathetic and sympathetic nervous systems. It brings heat and life, guaranteeing neurosensory balance. It controls excesses when there is an autonomic-nervous hyper-excitability. This meridian line, always in synergy with meridian line 36, contains and limits the metabolic impulse of the Liver/Gall Bladder family.

Stimulating This Meridian Line Improves the Biological Terrain in the Following Cases

In a psychological context:

apathetic temperament, with meridian line 36
lacking male expression, with meridian lines 36 and 06
to control neural balance, with meridian line 36
when one feels surrounded by the wrong crowd, with meridian lines 19 and 36
for better acclimating to the spring season, with meridian lines 11, 30, and 36

In a physical context:

in addition to treatments for congestive cerebral disorders, with meridian line 36
loss of sensitivity, with meridian lines 02 and 36
any phenomenon of plethora, with meridian line 30
thyroid gland problems, with meridian lines 36 and 27
flexibility of the skin, with meridian line 19

fragility of the elbow in men, with meridian lines 17 and 36
nasal discharge, with meridian lines 12 and 25
fragility of the shoulders in men, with meridian lines 05, 13, and 17
muscular coordination, with meridian lines 16, 36, 11, and 30
urinary problems, with meridian lines 22, 31, and 33
balance of the osseous frame, with meridian lines 18 and 17
filtration of waste, with meridian lines 30 and 01

Meridian Line 19 of Touch

Balances the Vital Currents of the Skin

This meridian line governs the overall balance of the skin (ectoderm, mesoderm, endoderm). The skin, with the hair, constitutes the organ governing the sense of touch, draws the silhouette of the body and plays the part of border between the internal world and the environment of our bodies. It is used as a filter when the organism is inundated in its functions of elimination.

Stimulating This Meridian Line Improves the Biological Terrain in the Following Cases

In a psychological context:

to feel at home in one's skin, with meridian line 03
tending to put oneself in other people's shoes, with meridian line 03
feeling of being surrounded by the wrong crowd:
- for women, with meridian lines 35 and 37
- for men, with meridian lines 36 and 38

In a physical context:

any cutaneous manifestation, often in conjunction with meridian lines 11 and 30, to assist prescribed medications
loss of flexibility in the skin, with meridian line 20
all capillary problems, with meridian line 03
flexibility of the skin:
- for women, with meridian line 37
- for a men, with meridian lines 38

lack of hydration, tonicity of the skin, with meridian line 22
all capillary problems, with meridian line 19
seborrheic hair (dandruff) with meridian lines 03, 11, and 30
skin with acne tendencies, with meridian lines 01 and 11

Meridian Line 03 of Potency

Balances the Vital Currents of the Hair

This meridian line controls the balance of the hair, whose sensitivity is influenced by sex hormones.

Stimulating This Meridian Line Improves the Biological Terrain in the Following Cases

In a psychological context:

to feel good in one's skin, with meridian line 19

tending to put oneself in other people's shoes, with meridian line 19

In a physical context:

all capillary problems, with meridian line 19

seborrheic hair (dandruff), with meridian lines 11, 19, and 30

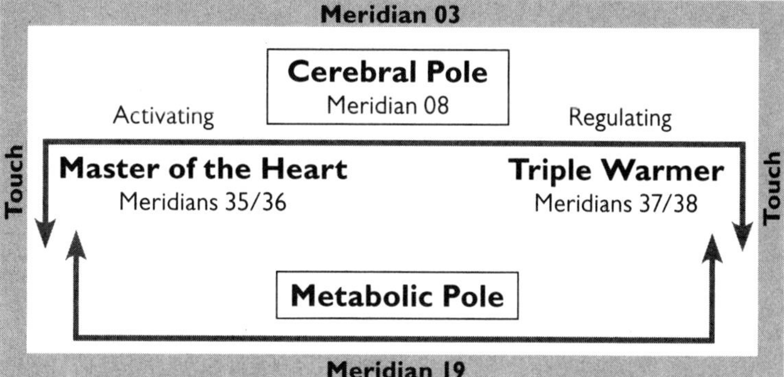

Fig. 8.9. The hair, skin, and sense of touch meridians

MERIDIAN LINES OF ORIENTATION: CONCEPTION AND GOVERNOR, THE TWO CENTRAL MERIDIAN LINES

Meridian Line 33 of Spatial Organization

Balances the Vital Currents of the Conception Vessel

The Conception meridian line is not associated with any specific organ. Its primary function, in synergy with meridian line 34

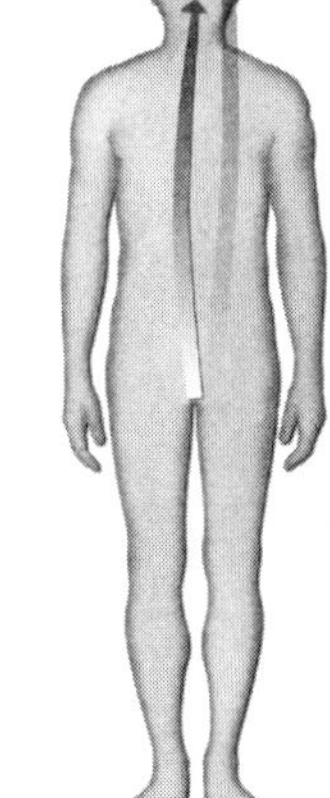

Fig. 8.10. The Conception and Governor lines connect the bottom and top halves of the body.

(Governor Vessel), is to connect the bottom and the top halves of the body, and to facilitate the communication between both the sexual and cerebral poles. This pair of meridian lines enables spatial recognition using the three planes of up–down, front–back, and right–left, in order to find your bearings.

Meridian line 33's specific activity supports "conception" on the mental and physical level: to conceive life, to realize and generate in accordance with the five senses.

Stimulating This Meridian Line Improves the Biological Terrain in the Following Cases

In a psychological context:

- lack of realization in one's life, with meridian line 18
- depressive tendencies, with meridian line 34
- to find desire (the taste) to live:
  - for women, with meridian line 28
  - for men, with meridian line 21
- difficulties of lateralization in the child, with meridian line 34
- spatial confusion, with meridian line 34

In a physical context:

- difficulties generating life:
  - for women, with meridian line 28
  - for men, with meridian line 21
- harmony of maternity (in women), with meridian lines 24 and 28
- urinary problems:
  - for women, with meridian lines 22, 37, and 31
  - for men, with meridian lines 22, 38, and 31
- contractions at the beginning of gestation, nausea, dislike (loss of the taste to give birth), with meridian lines 24 and 28
- stimulation of the gonads:
  - for women, with meridian lines 09, 29, and 35
  - for men, with meridian lines 09, 29, and 36
- digestive transit disorders, with meridian lines 05, 16, and 20
- postural balance, with meridian lines 16, 17, and 34
- acid reflux in the pregnant woman, with meridian line 10
- fatigue, with immune decline, with meridian lines 15 and 26

Meridian Line 34 of Spatial Orientation

Balances the Vital Currents of the Governor Vessel

Meridian line 34 is associated with no organ in particular, but its function is to connect, with meridian line 33, the bottom and top halves of the body and facilitate the communication between these two poles—sexual and cerebral. This pair of meridian lines enables spatial recognition, related to the three planes of a person: up–down, front–back, and right–left.

Meridian line 34 controls and directs the individual's vigor and allows him or her "to govern" his or her life.

Stimulating This Meridian Line Improves the Biological Terrain in the Following Cases

In a psychological context:

- lack of "personal control," too much creativity
- disorientated individual, with meridian line 33
- problems of lateralization in the child, with meridian line 33
- depressive tendencies, with meridian line 33

In a physical context:

- somnolence
- postural balance, with meridian lines 16, 17, and 33

A Brief Lexicon: Key Words of the Meridians

The five families of the meridians regulate the perception of the five senses, govern specific organ activities, and, depending on their vitality, bring about more or less coordinated behavior. We can better identify the impact of each family through key words, which can be spontaneously used for describing our moods and feelings. This makes it easier to grasp the role played by each meridian in the individual psychophysical dynamic.

Heart/Small Intestine Family • Sight • Summer

Meridian 04: Rhythm, Projection, Desire, Decision
Meridian 13: Choice, Selection
Meridian 01: Gift, Sharing
Meridian 32: Looking, Sight
Meridian 08: Attention, Integration, Elaboration

Stomach/Spleen-Pancreas Family • Taste • Late Summer/Seasonal Cusps

Meridian 10: Action, Work, Capacity
Meridian 18: Transformation, Respect
Meridian 21: Anchoring, Generation, Concretization, Male Realization
Meridian 28: Anchoring, Generation, Concretization, Female Realization
Meridian 17: Structuring
Meridian 26: Controlled, Centered Action

Lungs/Colon Family • Smell • Autumn

Meridian 20: Breath, Confidence, Expansiveness, Flexibility, Openness
Meridian 05: Organization, Hierarchical Ranking, Order
Meridian 25: Inspiration, Feeling
Meridian 12: Instinct, Intuition
Meridian 14: Virility
Meridian 24: Femininity
Meridian 06: Male Sexuality
Meridian 07: Female Sexuality
Meridian 16: Movement, Autonomy
Meridian 15: Self, Essence, Recognition, Immunity

Kidneys/Bladder Family • Hearing • Winter

Meridian 22: Assurance
Meridian 31: Alertness, Lucidity
Meridian 09: Vitality
Meridian 29: Receptivity
Meridian 02: Postural Balance, Verticality
Meridian 23: Representation, Visual Sensitivity
Meridian 27: Notion of Time, Being Present in the Moment

Liver/Gall Bladder Family • Touch • Spring

Meridian 11: Physical Energy, Serenity
Meridian 30: Calm, Forgiveness
Meridians 35–36: Intellectual Activity, Perception of One's Boundaries, Notion of Framework
Meridians 37–38: Neural Regulation, Perception of One's Boundaries, Notion of Framework
Meridian 19: Touch, Setting
Meridian 03: Connection, Prowess
Meridian 33: Spatial Orientation, Axis
Meridian 34: Spatial Orientation, Axis

PART THREE

Targeted Action with Sequential Nutripuncture

It's always the light that remains in the shadow.

EDGAR MORIN, *LE PARADIGME PERDU: LA NATURE HUMAINE*

9
Speaking the Language of the Body

THE ART AND THE MANNER

While the body is a vehicle to serve the human being, it also has its own biological life—it is living and lived in at the same time. Living fully means living in harmony with the body, tuned in to its language and perceptions, and its five senses that connect us to the world. Through this relationship, not always an easy one to manage, we can assert our tastes, be tuned in to ourselves and others, take advantage of our body's inspiration, and project its gaze over reality in order to finally feel "at home in our own skin."

However, an individual's particular sensibility can be influenced by events and other people. We have observed that certain situations can interfere with a person's taste, hearing, and vision, impinging on the integrity and balance of the cerebral cortex. The way a person acts and behaves then will be reactive, thereby altering his or her behavior and inducing physical and psychological irritation.

When a person is in harmony with her environment, she activates circuits that are compatible with her genetic potential and individual sensibility. Her meridians ensure cellular self-regulation, a balanced life dynamic, and consistent behavior. This person is fulfilled, and present to himself and others.

Conversely, if an individual is in conflict with his environment, he will activate reactive defense mechanisms, automatic responses that are sometimes incompatible with his particular sensibility, and therefore harmful to his vitality. This is how the information circulating in our bodies can interfere with the dynamic of the vital currents and have an adverse effect on our sensory and cognitive potential—in short, on the expression of our true personalities.

THE LANGUAGE OF THE MERIDIANS

Each meridian line communicates in its own way to contribute to the life of the organism (body). How is this language expressed? What are its codes? In this section of the book we will answer these questions by exploring the world of the information necessary for the equilibrium of organic complexity.

Our body, which connects us to the world, carries within it the knowledge of the evolution of life. It is an immense memory bank that is both cognitive (put together through personal experience) and biological (inherited through the genes). It is thanks to this transmission that our organism has evolved, by incorporating the information it needed to hone its functions and adapt to the environment. The human species passes this genetic legacy down from generation to generation. It carries various kinds of information, not only biological in nature but emotional and cultural as well, linked to the life experiences of our ancestors and the history of our civilization.

In addition to genetic information, the body also keeps a memory of emotional and sensory information connected with what we have experienced and which modulates the circulation of the vital currents. Like an enormous library, each of us has thousands of books at our disposal, with billions of pieces of information in our memory. This is real wealth that we can endeavor to learn to read so as to no longer remain hostages of our impulses (which in many cases are not truly ours), which interfere with the expression of our perception.

The gap existing between what we believe and the body's memory finds expression in perceptible modifications of the vital currents and the behavior they prompt. Sometimes all it takes is the mention of a traumatic incident to see a person in full health and composure suddenly plunge into a state of suffering triggered by his or her recall of what had been apparently forgotten emotions. This makes it possible to explain how the simple retention of an event can alter the current balance of the vital currents. Such memory can sometimes find expression in an upsetting way for people who have had organ transplants. They often exhibit the tastes, sensation, and even memories of the organ donor, demonstrating that this memory is quite real.

We have met people who repressed a traumatic event, who were absolutely positive it had been fully digested, classified, and even forgotten. In many cases, it only seemed to have been forgotten because the information was still active in their unconscious on the cellular level. All it took, in fact, was to ask them to retrace the circumstances of the event to see an immediate emotional change, sometimes accompanied by desperate weeping, which induced a change in specific vital currents (detected in the pulse). Conversely, people who have truly integrated a traumatic event cannot disrupt their vitality by evoking this stress: because the mind has integrated this event it is in agreement with the body and its memories. There are no inner conflicts between the body's reality and the individual's mental projections.

Where is this biological memory located? Is it on the hormonal cerebral plane or in the vital currents? It still remains a mystery. However, it has been seen that Nutripuncture, through its action on the circulation of the vital currents and stimulation of brain potential, helps integrate memories that might otherwise remain buried in our deepest depths like anti-personnel mines, where they reduce our vitality. It allows us to establish the necessary distance to confront them squarely, recognize their impact on our psychophysical equilibrium, and restore our optimal dynamic by "digesting" them.

Nutripuncture makes it possible for us to wake up our cognitive potential, enhance our self-awareness, and therefore distinguish between the information that can help us and the information we need to eliminate.

USING THE TWO NUTRIPUNCTURE APPLICATIONS

It is important to start with a simple Associative Nutripuncture approach (the General Cellular Nutritional Regulator plus the Nutris for the most weakened meridian lines) to stimulate the vitality of the organism before using Sequential Nutripuncture.

The purpose of Associative Nutripuncture is to mitigate the temporary difficulties challenging the individual so he or she can handle everyday stress and seasonal changes; this is done by nourishing the particularly disrupted circuits. All the meridian lines deemed necessary to reinforce the body's vital potential can be stimulated.

Associative Nutripuncture clears the cellular environment or terrain inside our bodies, boosting cellular exchanges and restoring a state of general well-being and vitality. It offers a full-spectrum stimulation through a very broad nutritional action. It has a regulating action, facilitating all biochemical exchanges and making it possible for each cell to extract the necessary nutrients for their proper function.

Sequential Nutripuncture, on the other hand, has a precise, targeted action that improves the depths of the biological terrain. It engages the body's language by connecting five specific meridian lines and stimulating them in a precise order. It communicates vital information that calls upon cellular organizational memory, enabling each meridian line to reposition itself correctly, recovering its proper place and function in the general structure of the body. The action of Sequential Nutripuncture is not limited to organic vitality but is quite broad and also promotes psychological and behavioral balance.

The principal goal of Sequential Nutripuncture is to optimize our cognitive potential while engaging fully integrated information at the cerebral level. It coordinates communication between peripheral circuits and the rhythmic activities in the cerebral pole. It offers a wide range of protocols for dealing with the stresses of life, which, from earliest childhood, have been weakening the vital currents. Sequential Nutripuncture must be properly targeted and well administered for full results to be seen.

In the following chapters of part 3, many specific applications of Sequential Nutripuncture are explained and the recommended sequences are listed. In keeping with the meridians' role in supporting the four vital parameters of the body discussed in chapter 3—bipolarity (positive yin-yang), fitting into a given space and time, spatial orientation, sensory and cognitive identity—applications of Sequential Nutripuncture include getting your bearings, discovering your body's potential, family dynamics, gender expression, coping with physical and psychological trauma, and supporting the body's structure and communication networks. In each case the protocol consists of ingesting a sequence of five Nutris corresponding to the numbers of the pertinent meridians. As mentioned earlier, these will vary for men and women when the meridians involved are those specific to each gender.

The language of the organism is that of the five elements. Nutripuncture communicates with the body by speaking this language. Each sequence of five Nutris is like a five-word sentence, a code that unlocks and activates something specific. The pills within the sequence are chewed and swallowed one at a time, paralleling how we hear each word in a sentence, one right after the other. Just like a meaningful sentence is not created by randomly placed words, the order of the nutriments must be respected in order to communicate properly with the organism. When a pair of Nutripuncture sequences is suggested, the first sequence is comprised of a specific sentence that connects five meridians and accesses cellular memory while the second sequence stimulates the cerebral pole to integrate and assimilate this cellular memory without disturbing any vital function. They are inseparable. The pills of both sequences are taken one after the other in succession.

For the organism to properly receive and learn the message, a given sequence (or pair of sequences) is usually taken twice a day for a month. However, just as with other kinds of learning, not everyone learns at the same rate and some require more review, so certain organisms may need additional time to learn the information. Occasionally, more than one sequence may be given to work on different levels of interactions that are the result of the vital currents not functioning properly.

The use of Sequential Nutripuncture for serious conditions requires a high level of understanding, which can be provided by a specialist who speaks this language of the body and can recommend the appropriate sequences.

Using Associative and Sequential Nutripuncture in the Same Day

You can use both Associative and Sequential Nutripuncture in the same day. However, it is recommended to let a period of at least two hours elapse between the times you take them. For example, if you are using the General Cellular Nutritional Regulator combined with other Nutris in the morning, it is a good idea to wait to take a sequence of complexes in the afternoon or, even better, the evening, so as to get the maximum benefit of their specific actions. Associative Nutripuncture has a dynamizing effect and Sequential Nutripuncture is relaxing.

10
Getting Your Bearings and Discovering Your Body's Potential

THIS CHAPTER EXPLORES the way you can find the right "phrase," the information that makes it possible to reconcile with your body, digest its memories, and discover good landmarks for joyfully moving ahead into the future.

The protocols offered here are generally suggested as an accompaniment to any kind of "personal development" approach, no matter what type (analytical, artistic, corporeal, and so on). They aid in addressing underlying blocks. Even when something is deeply desired and we strive ardently to apply ourselves, we are not always able to succeed. It is as if while driving we try to accelerate with the emergency brake on. Our deep wounds, over which we have constructed our defenses, resist the wished-for change, and the complexity of the reactions triggered on the cellular level are often difficult to disarm.

In such circumstances we usually continue working hard with our minds, omitting the life of the body and the memories that are buried in it like land mines. But still we remain stuck in place! The source of this frustration is countless pieces of information etched in our body's memory, which act as a dam, creating short circuits in our vital currents. This is the reason why so many people seek to escape their problems and flee reality by anesthetizing themselves in order to continue to live, or even survive.

The information that is etched in our memory began in utero and has been continuously evolving ever since, thanks to our life experiences. As we grow older, undergoing the countless transformations carrying us from embryo into adulthood, we still hold the previous ages in memory. Along the way, we can build ourselves or deform and destroy ourselves. Everything depends on the information we perceive, interpret, and integrate. It all plays a role in shaping the expression of our identity. This information does not always reach the conscious mind. It guides our actions and behaviors without our knowing, determining the biological terrain in which different disorders will appear.

In cases like this, Sequential Nutripuncture is of huge assistance. By encouraging the dynamic interplay of the circuits involved, it ensures the cognitive digestion and integration of information. This is essential for the construction of inner landmarks, getting our bearings, and expressing our sensory identity. Generally speaking, the majority of people who have put Sequential Nutripuncture to work in this way quickly realize its role in enabling them to:

- Face the memory of negative experiences
- Change harmful habits
- Change disagreeable reflexes
- Overcome multiple pitfalls that are preventing them from advancing

Constant Transformation in the Body

The most amazing quality of the body is its property of constant transformation. Thanks to its remarkable plasticity, all its cells evolve continuously. They evolve at different speeds depending on age, life quality, and the physiological and psychological state of the individual. In addition, in the same body completely different life cycles coexist: while the bone tissue entirely renews itself every five years and the cells of muscle tissue are renewed every seven years, those of the stomach and the skin live no more than three or four days. In the space of one lifetime thousands of generations of cells follow one another.

GETTING YOUR BEARINGS IN FIVE STEPS

The primary protocol offered by Sequential Nutripuncture fosters our ability to take charge of ourselves and integrate our body's lived experience on the cognitive level. This basic program of Sequential Nutripuncture makes it possible to strengthen and sometimes awaken specific circuits providing access to the information necessary to activate our vital potential. It is articulated in five stages, which make it possible to get our bearings and gradually discover our true potential in order to profit fully from life:

1. Asserting our existence
2. Acknowledging our genetic origin
3. Adopting our own body
4. Adopting our blood
5. Becoming aware of death and acknowledging the cellular cycle

Each of the five stages is worked on for an average of three or four weeks, at a rate of twice a day, depending on the individual's biological terrain and personal history.

First Step: Asserting Our Existence

Some of us have always known, deep down, that we were not the "fruit of love." Perhaps our parents had no desire for children and we were only born due to the chance occurrence of a sexual impulse capable of combining a sperm and ovum. Some of us were not truly wanted or acknowledged. Even if our parents did everything to keep us alive, they did not feed our desire to live or quench our thirst for love, the existential need of every child to feel welcome. But that no longer matters! We are here now, with an integral desire to live, which seeks expression, and our vital potential, although frozen or blocked, is only waiting to bloom.

Even if we have unconsciously adhered to this "projection of non-life," to this unconscious denial by our parents that made us feel miserably guilty about being in the world, it is still possible at any age to recognize and accept these facts and their influence over our childhood, and turn them to our advantage. This "negative" memory can become a strength, an excellent springboard for becoming a fulfilled, self-aware person, conscious of his or her potential, able to project a lucid and charitable gaze over his or her past.

Sequential Nutripuncture Protocol

This potential can be revealed by a protocol that stimulates these meridian lines in order: 07 or 06, 03, 33, 35 or 36, and 26.

After this first series, to encourage the integration of this information into the cerebral memory, a second series of meridian lines is stimulated: 30, 11, 04, 37 or 38, and 08.

Second Step: Acknowledging Our Genetic Origin

Over time, difficult communications with our parents, and tense and complex family dynamics can create an intolerable sense of discomfort, a deep conflict with our origins that we may sometimes wish to deny, erase, or even destroy. In fact, most of the time, our parents have cherished and nurtured us by projecting upon us their own emotional failings and existential difficulties. In cases like this, the activity of the Kidneys/Bladder family, related to the element of Water, can be greatly disrupted. A return to source, of an informational nature, is called for!

Acknowledging our origins involves deep acceptance, not only mental but cellular as well, of the sperm and ovum that gave us life. This recognition is a cognitive act that involves a certain self-awareness, an individual projection that allows us to find a place in life as the fruit of our parents (though without identifying with them). This calls on a potential that is often inhibited by a lot of stress, unrecognized by most of us and beyond our conscious awareness.

Sequential Nutripuncture Protocol

We can stimulate this potential by activating meridian lines: 15, 22, 37 or 38, 33, and 29.

Third Step: Adopting Our Own Body

We are adults and our body has been fully built. Even if it does not truly conform to what we would have wanted, it is the body we have. We therefore need to take ownership of our "fleshly property," inhabit it for the sake of experience, and learn to manage its potential, which in many cases, remains to be discovered. We need to cultivate it like a precious garden by awakening its full vitality. Respecting its needs, listening to its signals, learning its language, and calling upon its awareness are all part of establishing a healthy and authentic relationship with our self. To get a handle on our life and take charge of it, it is first necessary to adopt our body—living and lived in—the main headquarters of our identity and container of the sensations that awaken us to life.

Our relationship to our body, which we each experience in our own way, evolves over time through our physical and psychological maturation, shaped by our particular sensibility and by the kind of welcome we receive from our environment and the stimuli it offered us. It is completely natural for us to be one with our body if our parents: encouraged us as children to discover our own physical reality; acknowledged our creative gesture; and invited us to express our personal tastes, perspectives, and feelings, in short, our distinct sensory perception. But not all of us had the good fortune to grow up in welcoming surroundings, nor to receive all the stimuli we needed to learn and blossom. As adults, our relationship to our body is shaped by our education, culture, and experiences, especially our relationship with our mother.

Our relationship with our mother may still sometimes be fusional, that is, as if the umbilical cord joining mother and baby continued to exist, driving us to look for someone to play the role of mother. How many times have we been told "you'll always be my baby," a message that is etched so deeply in our body that few people can manage to freely experience their own bodies without feeling guilty. This prevents us from becoming autonomous and taking control over our own body in order to transform it in accordance with our individual codes.

But growing up means becoming autonomous and physically taking charge of ourselves. Even if we imagine ourselves to be a branch of the same tree, we still can allow ourselves to dwell freely in our own bodies; this is a completely natural process. No matter how old we are we can still refine our relationship to our body, find greater assurance, make our choices, and project ourselves into life guided by our own criteria for happiness.

Sequential Nutripuncture Protocol

For this purpose, stimulate these meridian lines in succession: 12, 09, 27, 22, and 29.

Fourth Step: Adopting Our Blood

When we are talking about the body, we are implicitly mentioning one of its most important components: the blood, which provides the energy every tissue needs to perform its activity. In addition to its role as nourishment, blood is also the symbol of the family bond, the element that allows the mother to feed the fetus throughout pregnancy.

Our blood's components are a mirror of our health. They are also the receptacle for countless bits of information, summarizing our individual development and history, the range of which we do not always grasp, though it can have such a profound effect upon our vitality.

Our blood, which was bequeathed us by our mother's womb, is today solely our personal property. Because of this, it is necessary to adopt it, just like our body, so we can put its energy—our energy—to better use to help transform and allow our body to live in harmony with its potential. To be capable of generating our own blood—which in the figurative sense is analogous to money—makes it possible for us to break from dependent relationships, especially those with our parents and other close friends and relatives. It also makes it possible to reinforce the biological terrain where circulatory disorders can appear, as well as the dynamics of the bloodstream in general.

Sequential Nutripuncture Protocol

We can stimulate in succession here the meridians 30, 01, 32, 13, and 37 or 38.

This extremely visceral information needs to be fully integrated on the cognitive level.

After this has been done, meridians lines 15, 04, 27, 34, and 08 can be stimulated.

Fifth Step: Becoming Aware of Death and Acknowledging the Cellular Cycle

To truly appreciate the value of life and give it meaning, it is essential to become conscious of death. "We live of death and die of life," said the Greek philosopher Heraclitus. Indeed, at every moment, hundreds of cells die while others are born: this is the cycle of life (fig. 10.1). Death nonetheless remains a mystery at the heart of existence and, according to Edgar Morin, "the problem that is more engrossing and puzzling than the origin of life, is that of the origin of death."[1] It can be asked if death may not be necessary to life.

Acknowledging death means seeing your reality in the life of the body, on the cellular level. Death is an inevitable aspect of life; it does not dominate us but is within us. It is through death that human beings find their characteristic humility that leads them to knowledge. Life then takes on its full meaning.

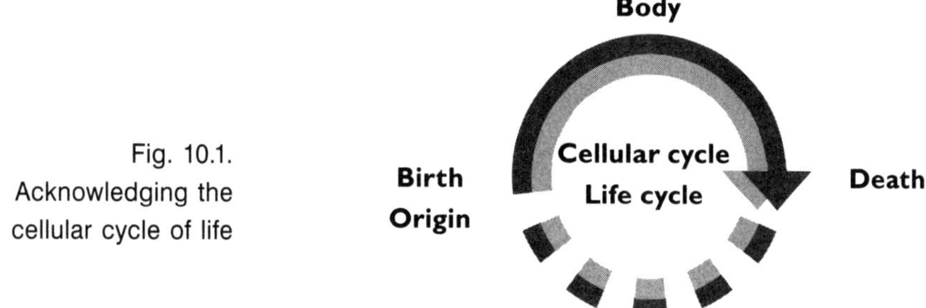

Fig. 10.1. Acknowledging the cellular cycle of life

The death of a beloved individual, recognized as a major stress, can be traumatic and induce a profound imbalance of the vital currents, one so extensive that it can create functional disorders and even illness. In the case of grief, we can experience this event differently—not by forgetting but by recognizing the deceased individual and the bond that we had. This is how we can transform an ordeal that is often difficult to overcome into an enriching experience, an opportunity for inner rebirth and a new start.

Sequential Nutripuncture Protocol

To encourage a better elaboration of the mourning process, we stimulate the following meridian lines in the indicated order: 26, 33, 04, 37 or 38, and 31.

PHASES OF HUMAN CONSTRUCTION

Human life is governed by a complex dynamic woven from the interaction of simple elements (cells) that organize together to give life to increasingly more sophisticated systems (organisms). This life is awakened by gradual stages that launch extraordinary "qualitative leaps" permitting the appearance of complex functions such as walking, language, thought, consciousness, and so forth. All abilities born from the emergence of new qualities that were not present at the level of the basic components can only appear in a context that is rich in sensory stimuli, both emotional and cultural.

Many years of research have shown that the qualitative leaps that mark off the human being's evolutionary phases awaken the vitality of specific meridians, which are more active at certain periods of life. These meridians carry vital impulses along their routes, which gradually increase our ability to interact with our context, stimulating qualitative leaps on the behavioral level and in tandem organizing increasingly complex brain functions.

When an evolutionary phase does not unfold harmoniously, for want of stimuli or because of an unfavorable environment, it can induce a disordered state of the individual's behavioral and social organization. Such disorganization is not often easy to offset in adulthood. Each stage must be fully realized for the succeeding stage to launch. If a stage is not fully realized, the evolutionary dynamic of the individual will lack the information required to mature emotionally, corporeally, and mentally, and hence to realize his or her potential. These evolutionary phases in the mental and physical maturation of a human being are shown in figure 10.2.

After birth three phases arouse the conditions necessary for building identity and communication:

Oral phase, which accompanies the gradual adaptation of babies to earthly life (stimulating the mouth and the sense of touch through the reflex movements of sucking and swallowing)

Anal phase, stimulating the learning process of intentional motility

Genital phase, the discovery of one's gender

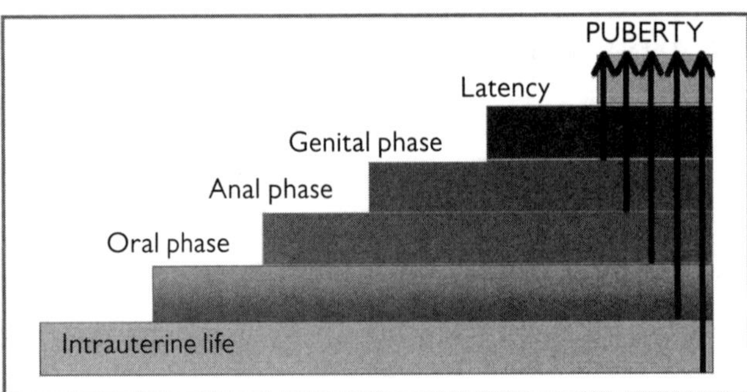

Fig. 10.2. Progressive interaction of the evolutionary phases

Nutripuncture has studied the full biological dimension of these three phases, not simply their psychological aspects. The oral phase awakens the ability to take possession of the energy needed by life and to articulate the sonorous codes of language, expressing openness, the power to take individual action, and body's capacity for change. The meridians associated with this stage are: 10/18 and 11/30.

The oral phase also paves the way for the anal phase, which is necessary to develop perception of the body's inner space. This period accompanies mastery of the muscles, intentional control of the sphincter and bladder, while awakening perception of the pelvis and, particularly, the organs of elimination. This phase ends when the child has become "potty trained," when he or she is able to easily master the movements involving contraction and dilation (the first level of motor coordination), expressing the ability to contain him or herself, in the broad sense of the term, heralding the first step of self-control. It accompanies internalization, the ability to sense one's own body (proprioception), and the perception of one's boundaries (skin and touch). The meridians that support the anal phase are: 22/31 and 20/05, along with and 35/37 for girls or 36/38 for boys.

The anal stage also prepares for the genital phase, which is characterized by the discovery of one's sex organs and one's identity as a boy or girl. It is the first contact with one's gender.

Numerous studies have shown that the first two phases of getting up to speed corporeally (both physically and mentally) are fundamental evolutionary moments in the blossoming of every individual during which the foundations for all future growth are laid down. Indeed, for a period of around thirty-six months, the child is learning how to manage the needs of the body, adjusting its impulses while savoring the sensations it offers and the pleasure of dwelling inside it. Normally, when these biological phases have been thoroughly played out, the genital phase benefits from all the energy that has been activated by all the meridians called upon for support during the oral and anal periods.

All forms of stress can hamper the smooth unfolding of these first two evolutionary phases, inhibiting the overall awakening of some vital currents and forming actual dams to their natural circulation. The rough draft of the inner landmarks necessary for the forming of identity will therefore be weakened, preparing a favorable terrain for the appearance of numerous psychophysical disorders. Once we have reached adulthood, in order to activate an often unexpressed vitality, it is beneficial to reinforce the dynamic of the circuits involved in the regulation of these first three evolutionary phases, which mark the construction of the foundations and essential bases for the expression of personal identity.

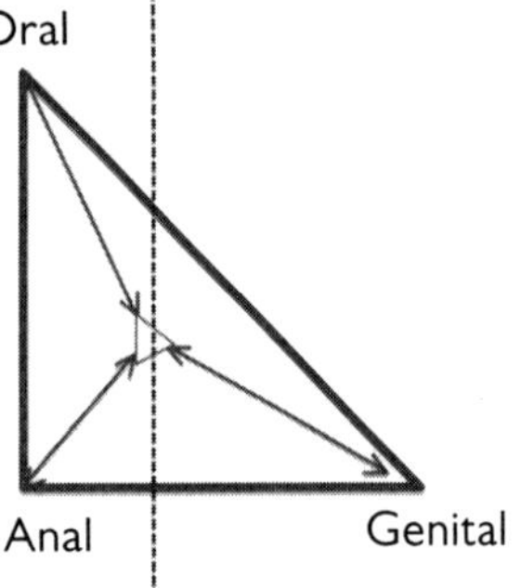

Fig. 10.3. Three foundations for the construction of the psychobiological human being

In fact, quite often, especially after becoming a parent, we are rudely tested by the resonance of the evolutionary phases of our baby on our own cellular memory. For example, the interaction established between the adult and a child going through the oral or anal phase can awaken old memories, going back to the times of our own childhoods. This may be deeply destabilizing and can trigger an emotional regression that is not always easy to manage.

We recall one Italian couple in particular who, after the birth of their first child, lost many of their personal benchmarks and fell into a sort of emotional vertigo that was triggered by their baby's entrance into his oral period. Stimulating the circuits involved in this phase allowed us to ensure a more tranquil parent-child dynamic, as well as offering the parents rich hindsight on their own experience as tiny children. This also allowed them to offer their child the presence of an upright man and woman solidly anchored to their foundations: the best evolutionary reference point for the growth of a child.

Nutripuncture enables people of any age to stimulate the meridian lines utilized in the activation of each "qualitative leap." This therapeutic method allows us to reactivate the phases lacking proper cellular integration and to desensitize the "scars" of childhood, still painful at any age. This will allow us to attain a sense of wholeness and the integrated expression of our own identity.

Sequential Nutripuncture for the Phases of Maturation

There is a specific sequential Nutripuncture protocol for each phase. We generally recommend starting with the oral phase because, as a primordial phase of getting up to speed with the body, it is indispensable. The Nutris for each phase should be continued twice a day for a month.

Oral Phase

Women: 18, 26, 30, 10, 11 + 05, 08, 12, 37, 02
Men: 18, 26, 30, 10, 11 + 05, 08, 12, 38, 02

Anal Phase

Women: 30, 05, 34, 07, 28 + 05, 04, 08, 26, 30
Men: 30, 05, 34, 06, 21 + 05, 04, 08, 26, 30

Genital Phase

Women: 35, 02, 33, 04, 37 + 31, 37, 28, 34, 26
Men: 36, 02, 33, 04, 38 + 31, 38, 21, 34, 26

How is this possible? There are so many different paths offered today that it can often be hard picking the one right for you! Furthermore, once committed to a particular path, you can often find yourself confronting a cellular memory that is so strong that it forms a dam to your awareness and your desire to increase your self-knowledge. Here Nutripuncture offers an excellent tool for learning the language of the body, reaching the deepest cores of our memory, and grasping their often paradoxical content. It makes it possible to access information often hidden from the mind, which can only be integrated on the cognitive level once the emotional and sensory routes have been opened and are ready to deliver their experience. In practice this approach can often restore the interrupted dialogue between mind and body. It encourages the awakening of sensory potential (often reduced if not outright anesthetized!) so that the cerebral cortex can consciously integrate the information captured from the environment.

11
The Family Dynamic and Gender Expression

THE INFORMATION CONTAINED in our familial context and parental relationships permits a child to implement the basic layers of personality and faculty of communication. If these foundations are not given suitable structure, some vital currents may be detoured away from their natural paths, thus forming a terrain that is favorable for the appearance of various disorders in adulthood. A child who receives the structuring information that is crucial for future development will gradually attain a certain sensory and cognitive maturity that will enable him or her to deal with the events of life without stress.

FAMILIAL TRIANGULATION

Every child positions him or herself as a boy or girl with respect to the parent couple. He or she naturally finds a place at the tip of a triangle with the mother and the father forming the base. The child generally has two reference frames: one provided by the parent of the same sex, the other by the parent of the opposite sex. When each parent lives in harmony with their individual reality as a woman or man (in other words without any ambivalence concerning their sexual identity) and plays their maternal or paternal role, the child (if his or her sexual identity is duly recognized) is automatically placed between these two opposite poles, yin-yang, without overly identifying with one or the other.

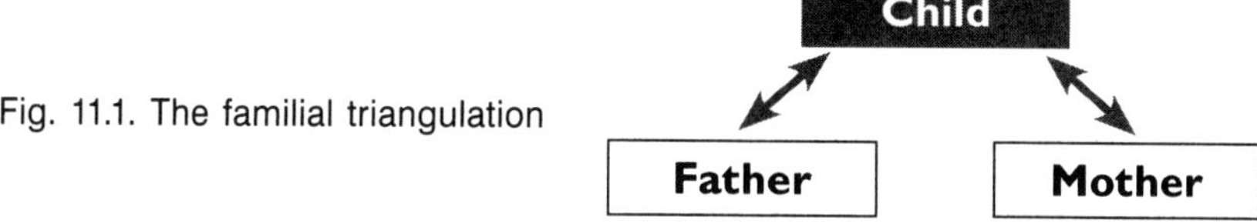

Fig. 11.1. The familial triangulation

However, a desire for fusion with the mother can linger as a remnant of the mutually beneficial, mother/baby symbiosis during the period from conception to weaning, which makes it possible for life to be given to a new being. In the behavioral development that marks the transition from the dyadic mother/baby relationship to the triadic dynamic of mother/baby/father, each of the three figures has their own place and role to play. At this stage the child generally displays an emotional projection toward the parent of the opposite sex. In psychoanalysis, this behavior is identified as the "Oedipus complex," which is recognized as an essential passage in the building of social relationships. Through this projection (which becomes visible between three and six or seven years of age), the child builds emotional reference points, sets standards and expectations for the other sex, and affirms his or her sexual reality.

At the age of reason, or at the latest during adolescence, a child is normally ready to move beyond this "complex." In fact, if the parent holds on, consciously or not, to the desire to form a couple with the child, this bond often becomes pathological, deforming the roles of each character in the family triangle and the overall behavioral dynamic.

Fig. 11.2. Familial triangulation: an important triadic dynamic

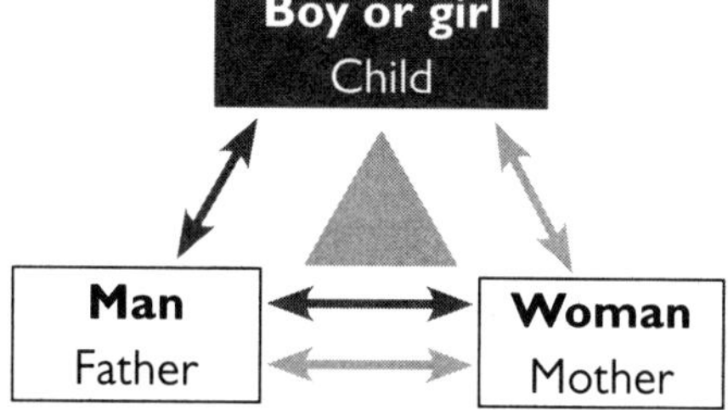

The Oedipus Complex: The Relationship with the Relative of the Opposite Sex

The standard description of the Oedipus complex focuses on the son's desire (conscious or unconscious) to seduce his mother: he cannot stand his father and wants to monopolize the attention of his mother. With daughters it is normally the other way around. Often this Oedipal relationship is obvious, but it also sometimes exists in a latent state.

Although the typical family structure has changed quite a bit in today's world—single parents and same sex parents are a reality—the Oedipal complex is an obligatory transition etched within human cellular memory. It is an archetype dwelling in the deepest regions of the mind. In some cases, it remains active during adulthood and can even persist for an entire lifetime, inducing behaviors that can affect romantic and family relationships. Sometimes, this Oedipal complex can emerge at the time of a new birth or can appear in a close attachment to a small child.

Based on the observations made in Nutripuncture research, an unresolved Oedipal attitude has an impact on the balance of several meridian lines: 04 (Heart), 30 (Gall Bladder), and 02 (Cerebellum). In adulthood the combined disruption of these three meridian lines is a "marker" of an unresolved Oedipus complex. The terrain this creates can spawn various disorders such as imbalances of lipids (fundamental constituents of the nervous system) and physical and psychological disorders (cardiac problems, extreme dizziness, gallstones, and so on).

Stimulating the vital currents of these meridian lines makes it possible to restructure a healthy relationship with one's parents (and children), to abandon infantile emotional projections, and to regain one's proper place and role in the family.

Sequential Nutripuncture Protocol

The following meridians should be stimulated to deal with this situation, in the order indicated: 04, 37 or 38, 34, 02, and 30.

After this first series, the following sequence of meridian lines should be stimulated: 32, 03, 37 or 38, 01, and 24 or 14.

Identifying with the Parent of the Same Sex: An Identity Trap

In family dynamics, the identification of the son with his father or the girl with her mother is a normal developmental progression of childhood, which can sometimes persist into adulthood. This identification, often revealed by a very profound mimetic attitude, is regarded as a natural consequence of affiliation.

However, when an individual goes through life relying on an external model, it insidiously induces disruptions of his or her ability to express a personal identity. This disturbs sensory perception, thereby weakening the individual's psychological and behavioral dynamic. Psychoanalysts define this pathology as a reversed Oedipus complex. In Nutripuncture, we have seen that this behavior is the primary factor in the manifestation of obsessive compulsive disorders (OCD); it also triggers serious alterations in the sense of smell.

The persistence of this identification with the father or the mother is more common than we might imagine. It is very probable that each one of us had to solve this fundamental problem of wanting to identify ourselves with the parent of the same sex. This desire is often fueled by the parent's behavior, which unconsciously adheres to the natural projections of the child, who, in his or her turn, relates to the parent's point of view. Stimulating the pertinent meridians at least once during your life will support your expression of personal identity and reinforce your male or female sensory perceptions.

Sequential Nutripuncture Protocol

Begin with the following meridian lines: 12, 09, 18, 37 or 38, and 08.

After this first series, the second series to be stimulated should be this sequence of meridian lines: 02, 24 or 14, 12, 30, and 08.

Acknowledging Your Father and Mother to Better Position Yourself as a Daughter or Son

In the family triangle, two essential aspects need to be recognized and integrated. The first relates to the independent expression of the traditional three main players of the family unit: the man and the woman, in their reciprocal relationship of mutual recognition, and the child, girl or boy, as an individual containing all the potential of the adult he or she will grow up to be.

The second aspect relates to the maternal and paternal role in which the couple has been invested since conception. Every couple with children has connected to the evolutionary line of humankind, and to its genetic memory and relational experience, which has been honed and refined for thousands upon thousands of years. By the same token, a couple allows a third character, the child, to fit into this evolutionary chain.

Becoming aware of one's paternal or maternal role in the evolutionary line of humanity is what makes it possible to acknowledge one's child as a son or a daughter. More importantly it allows parents to create a healthy distance from their child, by offering themselves to be like a bow with which the child projects him or herself forward into life, without fusion or possession. In short, this manifests what the poet Khalil Gibran wrote about children: "they do not belong to us, they arrive through us; they are children of life." This enables the child, completely naturally, to assume the role of son or daughter to each parent, as well as to recognize him- or herself, along with his or her progenitors and ancestors, as links in the long chain of human affiliation, without any fusion or identity confusion.

In Nutripuncture it has been verified that when a person has deep conflicts about their parents, and therefore an unconscious refusal to belong to the chain of affiliation, different vital currents will deviate from their proper course. It would appear that many allergy problems (such as to lactose, gluten, pollens) can develop in this terrain.

After stimulating the meridian lines involved here with a specific Sequential Nutripuncture protocol, we can better situate ourselves as a son or daughter, with regard to our mother and father, and feel this broader connection with the human evolutionary line to which we all belong. This is why some practitioners often prescribe the sequence below for children who have trouble asserting themselves or finding their true place with respect to their parents.

If you have been adopted and do not know who your biological parents are, you can use this same protocol for strengthening your own feelings of belonging to the chain of affiliation.

Sequential Nutripuncture Protocol

Affiliation

For women: 27, 09, 37, 02, 04 + 30, 13, 34, 27, 08

For men: 27, 09, 38, 02, 04 + 30, 13, 34, 27, 08

Role

Maternal: 26, 02, 33, 37, 12 + 08, 12, 04, 11, 28

Paternal: 08, 38, 32, 16, 30 + 08, 36, 03, 32, 38

GENDER ADOPTION OR REJECTION

Fully expressing sexual characteristics—male or female—is fundamental for psychological and physical balance. From birth, girls and boys have completely different body types, due to their specific sex organs, which are located inside for girls and outside for boys. The energy that each projects is also very distinctive: that of girls is more receptive, and of boys is more projective. This sexual energy gradually evolves after birth according to the stimuli of the environment.

Sexual Energy

In Nutripuncture, when we speak of sexual energy, we are referring to the existential impulse, the vital force that animates a baby from its very youngest age, rather than the sexual activity he or she engages in later after puberty.

The oral phase of development (see chapter 10) awakens and channels the existential impulse of the nursing-age child, conferring a major erogenous role upon his or her mouth. Next, the activity of the sphincters (anal and vesical) make it possible to learn muscle control (this is when the first intentional movements occur) and pave the way for the genital stage. Puberty, the ultimate objective of this process of sexual maturation, is completed at adulthood in tandem with cognitive maturation.

In adulthood, the expression of our sexuality is often shaped by the conditions of the family circle, which have also determined the way we experience and handle our bodies. The unconscious desire of the parents concerning the sex of their child can disturb the expression of the child's male or female polarity, which manifests during adolescence. When a conflict or an outright denial of personal gender exists, and if the individual wishes to address this, a specific Sequential Nutripuncture protocol is available.

Sequential Nutripuncture Protocol

For women, the circulation of the meridian lines involved in the expression of one's femininity can be invigorated in this order: 35, 24, 27, 07, and 12.

After this first series has been worked, a second series of meridian lines can be stimulated: 27, 15, 29, 35, and 07.

For men, the circulation of the meridian lines involved in the expression of virility can be regulated: 36, 14, 27, 06, and 12.

After this first series has been worked, a second series of meridian lines can be stimulated: 27, 15, 29, 36, and 06.

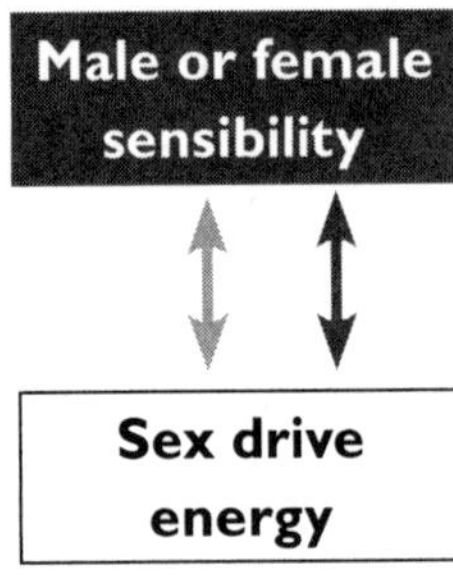

Fig. 11.3. The relationship between gender expression and sex drive impulses

Expressing Your Femininity or Virility in Adulthood

In Nutripuncture when we speak about polarity, we are referring to a yang energy (virility) and a yin energy (femininity), which manifest quite openly during puberty. This sensitivity is quite different from the sex drive impulses (male and female) present since birth. The appearance of the secondary sex organs (breasts for young girls or Adam's apple for young boys) cements the puberty stage, which is now quite visible in the upper part of the body and offers access to another psychological level of expression.

Normally during adulthood, it is the upper part of the body that regulates the impulses of the lower part of the body; this polarity regulates the sexual expression of the individual, governed by meridian line 06 (Penis) or 07 (Vagina). Puberty is a fundamental passage, activating inborn information that is necessary for human sexuality and for stimulating the interactions between pelvis/shoulders, sexuality/polarity, and impulse/integration. People who have had bad experiences during this period or who quite simply refuse to acknowledge this life change (going so far as actually rejecting their sex organs), often exhibit major behavioral disorders related to the deviation of the various families of meridian lines.

You can acknowledge your femininity or virility by activating the meridian lines that have been most weakened. This is a basic step to living in harmony with your sexual body, a source of fulfillment for the mind and vital well-being for the body, and the foundation for establishing an essential identity landmark.

Sequential Nutripuncture Protocol

For women, we can invigorate the circulation of the following meridian lines: 25, 15, 33, 37, and 07.

Following this first series, stimulate this series of meridians next: 05, 12, 07, 08, and 33.

For men, the circulation of the following meridian lines can be invigorated: 25, 15, 33, 38, and 06.

Following this first series, stimulate this series of meridians next: 05, 12, 06, 08, and 33.

If erectile dysfunction exists, this stimulation has proven itself extremely helpful, especially when used to supplement the Associative Nutripuncture protocol in which the General Cellular Nutritional Regulator is combined with activation of meridian lines 06, 14, and 36. You can use the Associative Nutripuncture protocol in the morning and the Sequential Nutripuncture protocol in the evening.

The Breasts

For women, their breasts are receptors of their femininity. However, their balance can be put to the test, depending on how they adopt or refuse the path that leads to their lives as women. Diet, hormonal secretions, sex life, and a good number of other elements can influence breast balance, which can be the site of numerous disorders, especially for those women who are fifty years or older.

Sequential Nutripuncture Protocol

To help a woman to better express the power of her femininity as exemplified by her breasts, the meridians that govern this expression can be stimulated: 29, 15, 27, 24, and 09.

After this first series, a second series of meridian lines can be stimulated: 24, 33, 04, 08, and 32.

The Adam's Apple

Once puberty kicks in, the larynx of the young boy changes: under the influence of hormones the thyroid cartilage adopts the shape of a shield. The boy's voice changes and becomes deeper in tone. If a man has a hard time asserting himself or expressing virility through his voice, the following Sequential Nutripuncture protocol will allow him to assert his virility, display his polarity, and better express his sexual nature.

Sequential Nutripuncture Protocol

The following meridian lines can be stimulated: 36, 01, 04, 15, and 14.

Following this first series, a second series of meridian lines can be stimulated: 01, 32, 14, 08, and 38.

Menopause

Menopause is a profound change of a hormonal nature that enables the woman to reach a new dimension of herself and makes it possible for her femininity to bloom in its deepest and most essential fashion. However, this is a complex transition—a true metamorphosis—that is fairly long and accompanied by several annoying factors. The halt of ovarian function severs the communication between the gonads and hypothalamus, and as hormone production becomes more erratic, it causes hot flashes and vaginal dryness. The vital currents, which already existed in a latent state before puberty, will gradually shape a new hormonal dynamic appropriate for a new season of life in the body.

Menopause has a very strong impact on a woman's body clock, especially on the thyroid and its meridian line, which governs time. In this period of a woman's life, Nutripuncture has proven effective as a very valuable "bodyguard" for offering general relief from the irritating symptoms that accompany menopause. It offers a means of invigorating the most weakened meridians in order to adjust (before, during, and after menopause) hormonal fluctuations and restore complete vitality.

Sequential Nutripuncture Protocol

The meridians on which the heaviest demands are made during menopause, and therefore require stimulation, are: 28, 27, 16, 31, and 34.

After this series, the second series to be stimulated are: 05, 27, 08, 31, and 23.

12
Coping with Physical and Psychological Trauma

ONCE WE HAVE ADOPTED our sexual body and our male or female polarity has been integrated, we are at long last qualified to assume command of this "vehicle/body." We are now physically capable of controlling our bodies/selves in a way that allows us to fully experience life as well as governing the impact of that experience on our psychophysical balance.

However, we have seen that certain stresses and traumas can exceed the self-regulation capacities of our organism and weaken specific circuits, to the point of interfering with our psycho-emotional balance. This is what happens when people, disturbed by their environment, lose control of their body and can no longer manage to express themselves in harmony with their identity. Here, Sequential Nutripuncture plays a significant role by stimulating the overworked circuits thus affected or even exhausted.

THE EVENTS OF LIFE: STRESSORS OR STIMULI?

Nutripuncture makes it possible to deal with the various forms of stress most of us encounter in life, although we are not always aware of the impact they are having on our vitality. It is only after we have restored drive to the most weakened vital currents that we can truly evaluate their burden and realize the extent of the pain and discomfort we were carrying. Many clinical observations over a period of several years have made it possible to decode the body language linked to critical life experiences and locate the meridian lines implied in the psychophysical management of certain events, a few of which are described here.

Divorce: A Physical Separation

Marriage, whether civil, religious, or a simple union, deeply engages each partner in its success and involves key behavioral modifications. Thus, in the event of separation or divorce, it has been seen that certain bonds, products of the "hooked atoms" that allowed the classic "love at first sight" phenomenon, usually become difficult to break, making it difficult for a person to find individual freedom and psychophysical autonomy.

Divorce can be a traumatizing experience even if in certain cases it can appear to be liberation. It has been shown that there will always be a cellular memory of the bonds created between the two people, based on the behavioral system they maintained during their relationship. It is therefore important to reinforce the circuits that were most affected during this time in order to recover one's own identity reference points and freedom.

In order to integrate this separation on the emotional and cognitive levels and recover some kind of serenity, the meridians involved in this kind of experience and often weakened by it can be given support. The people who have employed the following protocol have described it as helping them to turn an apparently negative experience to their advantage. Once the impact on the vital currents was integrated, it became beneficial and gave them what they needed to really make a "new start."

Sequential Nutripuncture Protocol

For women: 30, 09, 22, 15, 33 + 17, 37, 11, 32, 33

For men: 30, 09, 22, 15, 33 + 17, 38, 11, 32, 33

Suicide

The suicide of a loved one is experienced completely differently than a natural or accidental death. Scarring on specific meridian lines can be seen, which has a particular impact on the mental level. Those who have tried to commit suicide, as well as those who have lost a loved one to suicide or witnessed a suicide, suffer a disruption of the fundamental flow of their vital currents. The memory of this action, recorded at the cellular level, runs the risk of coming back to the surface at the time of a severe stress. The information it reactivates can be hard for the cerebral cortex to control.

Sequential Nutripuncture Protocol

The following meridians lines can be invigorated in order to disarm a pain, sometimes deeply buried, which is gaining the upper hand over our desire to live:

For women: 33, 37, 11, 02, 34 + 09, 08, 17, 02, 11

For men: 33, 38, 11, 02, 34 + 09, 08, 17, 02, 11

Abortion: A Stress that Is Often Repressed

Abortion is always a challenging event, even if there is every reason in the world to go through with this procedure. It is understandable why a woman, facing the hardships of life and the choices it imposes upon her, can choose abortion, as this is sometimes the only solution imaginable. No matter the motive (good or bad), it always leaves a deep wound at the cellular level, where hidden pain remains in a latent state for years, preventing the woman from fully living life to the fullest extent. Certain women even manage to completely repress this event from their memory, but it is only temporary, since it is ultimately important to recognize it and "digest it" at the cellular level.

Sequential Nutripuncture Protocol

The following meridians can be stimulated in this order: 28, 22, 33, 26, and 12.

After this first series, the second series of meridian lines to stimulate is: 19, 27, 02, 08, and 03.

Rape: One of the Most Devastating Traumas

In body language, rape is experienced as a vicious attack to one's integrity, which affects the skin, our physical and sensory "frontier." Sometimes other seemingly minor events can be perceived as an assault, causing psychological violence and humiliation. Even if the victim is conscious of the psychophysical repercussions of this event, its emotional, moral, and physical burden always remains in memory.

Subconsciously, to protect themselves from the shock, people can block all thought of a traumatic event, although it remains etched in their cellular memory. To restore their lost integrity, it is necessary to restore the circuits that were disrupted by this act of denial.

Sequential Nutripuncture Protocol

For women, this order of meridian lines should be stimulated: 35, 33, 07, 03, and 37.

Once this is done, the following meridian lines can then be stimulated: 03, 24, 02, 08, and 07.

For men, this order of meridian lines should be stimulated: 36, 33, 06, 03, and 38.

Then the following meridian lines can be stimulated: 03, 14, 02, 08, and 06.

Memory of a Trauma

The cellular memory of an accident can also affect our overall dynamic, causing a general disordered state of our organism and inducing various diseases. Each time the body undergoes a physical shock (such as a car accident or a fall), even if it is an old event, valuable information circulating at the time of the accident remains fixed in memory, especially at the bone level. This disrupts the biological rhythms and the individual's temporal anchoring, essential ingredients for our vitality.

Invigorating the circuits weakened by the trauma promotes the integration of this information to find a better structural balance, at the physical and psychological level. This encourages the individual's ability to anchor him or herself in his or her personal space and time.

Sequential Nutripuncture Protocol

For women: 17, 27, 09, 37, 34 + 16, 12, 27, 02, 17

For men: 17, 27, 09, 38, 34 + 16, 12, 27, 02, 17

Remorse and Forgiveness

True forgiveness is very often the hardest thing in the world to achieve because, at the cellular level, we are not always able to "move on." In certain cases, the reaction can be very violent: "To forgive? Never! I'd rather die." On the other hand, many people have the impression they have forgiven another person or themselves, but this is often an illusion, as the information has not really been circulated through the corresponding circuits. Their impression is a purely intellectual, mental projection.

The stimulation of disrupted vital currents enables us to become aware of our festering wounds and to find certain serenity in attaining cellular forgiveness. When the meridians that govern the feeling of humility have been properly regulated, cellular forgiveness can indeed be obtained. This alleviates latent agony, which can stick to an individual throughout their entire life, condition troubled behavior, and lay the foundations for psychosomatic disorders.

Sequential Nutripuncture Protocol

For women: 37, 23, 04, 12, 11 + 26, 03, 34, 23, 32

For men: 38, 23, 04, 12, 11 + 26, 03, 34, 23, 32

13
Supporting the Body's Structure and Communication Networks

THE LIVING STRUCTURE OF THE BODY

Bone, muscle, and skin are three interactive elements that allow the body to move in space (fig. 13.1). These three systems are not isolated, but fully connected with the overall dynamic of the body. Each has its own function, is animated by different communication circuits, and occupies a particular place in the spatial organization of the body:

The skeleton is the most internal element, which provides the framework for the muscles.
The muscles, located between the skin and bones, are the engines for our actions.
The skin that envelops us forms the interface between the outer surroundings and our inner world.

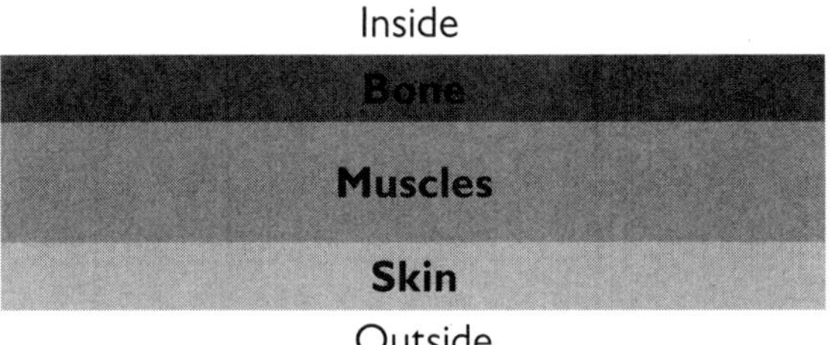

Fig. 13.1. The three interactive elements that allow the body to move

Every physical trauma has an impact on the circulation of the vital currents and can detour the information that ensures the balance of our frame (skeletal, muscle, and tactile) creating a biological terrain in which physical and psychological disorders can take root, troubles that may resist identification.

The Skeletal Structure

Bone pain often represents a transformation process of the tissues, which in turn are no longer receiving enough of the necessary information to activate self-regulation. Often, individuals with these problems experience spatial confusion, affecting the organization of their body diagram and thus slowing down their general motor coordination.

Whether for the growing child, the athlete, the menopausal woman, or the elderly, Sequential Nutripuncture can support general structural balance, reinforce the state of well-being, and harmonize previously choppy movements. The sequence given here is also advised for people with their "heads in the clouds," who lack balance and concentration.

Sequential Nutripuncture Protocol

For women: 35, 15, 17, 11, 30 + 02, 34, 26, 17, 27

For men: 26, 15, 17, 11, 30 + 02, 34, 26, 17, 27

The Teeth: Mirror of Each Individual's Life Experience

While teeth are not bones per se they are considered part of our skeletal system. Studies by dental researchers have made us consider teeth as the "fuses" of an electrical circuit: the vitality of each tooth depends in fact upon the meridian that regulates it. When a problem appears there is always an underlying disturbance, connected with the circuit that feeds it. Any disruption (physical, functional, or psycho-behavioral) interfering with the circulation of the meridian lines can cause postural alterations—an imbalance in the jaws and the teeth. The effect of Nutripuncture on complex postural alterations has been measured, thanks to various tests (podoscope, podograph, goniometry, and so forth). Dental research has shown that when the circuits related to a disrupted dental area are stimulated, its terrain is drained; then the tooth is given greater resistance to cavities and the gums will have less tendency to recede.

Following a dental treatment, a targeted Nutripuncture treatment will spur on the self-regulating systems and increase tolerance to the materials used by the dentist. From a simple cavity to a more complex implant, less regressions and complications have been seen after treatment, as well as a more rapid adaptation by the patient to the new arrangement in his or her mouth.

If a tooth is prepped before surgery, by providing it with information that will "feed" its biological terrain, there will be better response from the tissue, greater pain tolerance, less bleeding, and therefore less stress for the patient; the procedure will also be less taxing for the doctor.

In orthodontics, a targeted Nutripuncture treatment stimulates the harmonious growth of the jawbones and encourages the performance of braces and other dental appliances. Problems concerning uncoordinated movement of the tongue, pharynx, and face, observed in both children and adults and connected with a variety of factors such as mouth breathing, thumb sucking, and sucking on the tongue, bottle feeding, and so forth, have been resolved in 85 percent of the people who have stimulated the recommended circuits.

Sequential Nutripuncture Protocol

For women: 33, 16, 35, 27, 10 + 33, 28, 26, 16, 10

For men: 33, 16, 36, 27, 10 + 33, 21, 26, 16, 10

The Muscle Structure

All the meridian lines take part in the overall dynamic of the muscle system, each offering the muscles a distinct quality:

- Stomach/Spleen-Pancreas pair: Strength
- Kidneys/Bladder pair: Tonicity
- Lungs/Colon pair: Flexibility
- Heart/Small Intestine pair: Impulse
- Governor/Conception and Master of the Heart/Triple Warmer pairs: Motor Skills
- Liver/Gall Bladder pair: Metabolic Regulation; Healthy Energy Flow

To ensure the balance of the skeleton, it is important to jointly stimulate the circuits of the skeletal and muscle systems. Especially for athletes, after having

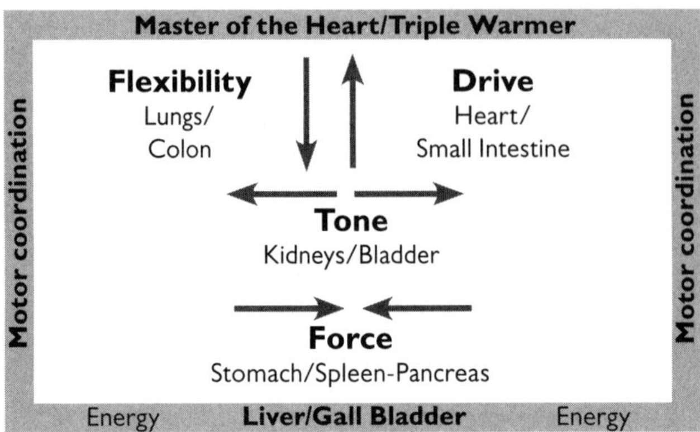

Fig. 13.2. Movement properties and the meridians involved

"fed" the meridians of the skeletal structure, these next circuits should be regulated in order to ensure optimal muscle dynamics.

Sequential Nutripuncture Protocol

For women: 16, 37, 31, 18, 30 + 16, 08, 33, 26, 02

For men: 16, 38, 31, 18, 30 + 16, 08, 33, 26, 02

Sports: Avoiding Aches and Cramps

Practicing any sport can make huge demands on the bone/joint and muscular systems. This can cause aches or cramps, often connected to a lack of practice, nutritional deficiencies, or poor elimination. A Sequential Nutripuncture protocol is recommended for all athletes to reduce the side effects of sports and optimize the balance of the meridians on which the greatest demand is placed by athletic effort.

Sequential Nutripuncture Protocol

Used before and after exercise, this sequence for both women and men encourages rapid recuperation after training or a match: 16, 27, 18, 15, 22.

The Skin Structure

Skin exhibits different characteristics depending on what part of the body it covers. It is a genuine mirror of our internal functions and helps in the determination of precise pressure points, whose sensitivity signals that the corresponding meridian lines require regulation. The expression of "feeling good in your skin" means that the boundaries of the individual are well defined, enabling him or her to interact in an optimal way with his or her surroundings.

The condition of the skin is dependent upon the harmonious interaction of two poles: the metabolic and neural centers. The first governs the underlying metabolism; the second ensures the skin's projective glow, its radiance. The drainage of the skin, in particular the subcutaneous cellular tissue, depends upon the underlying lymphatic system.

Sequential Nutripuncture Protocol

To nourish the overall balance of the skin, the following sequence of vital circuits can be invigorated:

For women: 19, 27, 03, 08, 33 + 19, 32, 08, 33, 34

For men: 19, 27, 03, 08, 33 + 19, 32, 08, 33, 34

Warts? Competition Between Skin Layers

The skin consists of three layers: ectoderm, mesoderm, and endoderm. An outbreak of warts betrays an imbalance of the information conveyed by the meridian lines that feed these three layers.

Sequential Nutripuncture Protocol

For women: 34, 31, 37, 33, 22 + 12, 15, 03, 19, 08

For men: 34, 31, 38, 33, 22 + 12, 15, 03, 19, 08

The Subcutaneous Cellular Tissue

This is a tissue that plays the role of shock absorber; it is what gives skin its tension. This tissue supports the skin, hydrates it, and nourishes it. Stimulating the meridian lines in connection with this tissue promotes tonicity in tired and sagging skin. This Sequential Nutripuncture protocol is very helpful, especially for people over fifty, in maintaining the overall tone of the tissues.

Sequential Nutripuncture Protocol

For women: 35, 19, 24, 15, 03 + 05, 02, 12, 15, 19

For men: 35, 19, 14, 15, 03 + 05, 02, 12, 15, 19

The Mucous Membranes

The mucous membranes cover all the internal cavities and ensure proper lubrication of the tissues. In the event of excessive secretions at the pulmonary, vaginal, or other levels, one can regulate the discharge by invigorating the following meridian lines.

Sequential Nutripuncture Protocol

For women: 19, 20, 26, 37, 33 + 03, 08, 24, 16, 19

For men: 19, 20, 26, 38, 33 + 03, 08, 14, 16, 19

Hair

Our hair is a mirror of our vitality. Stress, a poor diet, and harsh weather conditions are all factors that can weaken it. Some parts of the scalp are particularly sensitive to hormones, causing—especially in men—an increasing loss of hair. Stimulating the circuits governing the self-regulation of the hair will not restore a full head of hair but it will fortify what is left by restoring its strength and vitality.

Sequential Nutripuncture Protocol

For women: 03, 27, 31, 22, 37 + 03, 08, 01, 32, 02

For men: 03, 2,7 31, 22, 38 + 03, 08, 01, 32, 02

The Mucous Membrane-Skin-Hair Dynamic

If there are disorders pertaining to mucous membranes, skin, and hair, you should always look for a disruption in the circulation of the Master of the Heart and Triple Warmer meridian lines. The latter in particular plays a role in maintaining neuro-sensory balance, which controls all excesses in the event of neuro-vegetative hyperexcitability. The synergistic function of these meridian lines can be nourished with a specific Sequential Nutripuncture protocol, which invigorates their connections in the meridian line network.

Sequential Nutripuncture Protocol

Concerning the balance of the Master of the Heart:

For women: 04, 32, 35, 33, 02 + 29, 02, 01, 35, 33

For men: 04, 32, 36, 33, 02 + 29, 02, 01, 36, 33

Concerning the balance of the Triple Warmer:

For women: 33, 11, 13, 37, 02 + 12, 02, 26, 19, 27

For men: 33, 11, 13, 38, 02 + 12, 02, 26, 19, 27

SUPPORTING THE MERIDIANS THAT ENSURE THE DYNAMIC OF THE BODY'S MAJOR COMMUNICATION NETWORKS

As we grow older, we need to give thought to the regular maintenance of the body's major communication networks and support the meridian lines governing their circulation. The third leading cause of death (after heart attacks and cancer) in the United States is stroke. It is the second leading cause of death in the Western world. We can ask if there is a preexisting condition for this, or if it simply reflects the lack of maintenance given the vital currents concerned? It is obvious to us that such conditions arise from a biological terrain; therefore we must take pains to reinforce the circulation of the currents involved.

The information circulating in meridian line 01 (secondary circuit in the Heart/Small Intestine family), which carries blood into the organs, is of a projective nature. Conversely, meridian line 29 (secondary circuit in the Kidneys/Bladder family) is of a receptive nature, ensuring the return of the blood charged with the information of cellular experience.

While the heart is the engine that drives the blood's movement, the arteries cause it to circulate, and the veins carry it back to the heart. On the psychological level the round trip is expressed by the capacity of giving (arteries) as well as receiving (veins). Any "informational" imbalance between the artery system and the vein system can induce, over the long term, circulatory disorders. Encouraging the dynamic of the meridian lines involved here puts the communication between the functions of projection and reception back in tune.

The lymphatic system is governed by meridian 15 of the Lungs/Colon family. If, by way of an illustrative example, we were to say that the artery corresponds with the intake and the vein with the return of the metabolic transformation that takes place on the cellular level, we could say that the lymphatic system is responsible for the circulation of the cell's "perspiration," the essence released by its metabolism, its distillate and perfume.

We recommend the use of a specific Sequential Nutripuncture protocol for invigorating the networks involved in arterial, vein, and lymphatic communication for everyone over fifty. This upkeep is especially advisable for people with poor blood circulation, and should be performed once a year.

Sequential Nutripuncture Protocol

It is always a good idea to jointly regulate the activity of the meridians related to the arteries and veins, as their harmonious interaction is essential for overall good blood circulation.

To regulate the meridians involved in arterial projection, stimulate:

For women: 01, 34, 04, 08, 32 + 37, 11, 01, 08, 02

For men: 01, 34, 04, 08, 32 + 38, 11, 01, 08, 02

To regulate the meridians involved in vein receptivity, stimulate:

For women: 29, 09, 33, 35, 23 + 30, 15, 35, 29, 08

For men: 29, 09, 33, 36, 23 + 30, 15, 36, 29, 08

To support the meridians involved in lymphatic circulation, the following circuits should be invigorated:

For women: 25, 15, 33, 24, 07 + 25, 05, 15, 12, 13

For men: 25, 15, 33, 14, 06 + 25, 05, 15, 12, 13

This protocol strengthens immune defenses and has proven quite to helpful for convalescents, very young children, and the elderly. It is also helpful to use this protocol before a lymphatic draining in order to invigorate the lymphatic currents and optimize the benefits of the massage.

14
Sequential Nutripuncture of the Five Families and the Five Senses

THE FIVE FAMILIES of meridians introduced earlier are here examined from the Sequential Nutripuncture perspective, which makes it possible to restore each "member" of the family to its proper place and function in the body's dynamic, at full potential.

THE STOMACH/SPLEEN-PANCREAS FAMILY

Reminder: These meridian lines make it possible to enter and build our life. They govern the sense of taste and translate the nurturing capacities of Earth, making it possible to feed and build a healthy body.

In the circadian cycle, the meridian line of the Stomach is more active between 7 a.m. and 9 a.m. Then, the circulation of the Spleen-Pancreas meridian line takes over and becomes more sustained between 9 a.m. and 11 a.m. Normally, the circulation of the Stomach meridian line activates that of the Pancreas, as it is action that leads to realization and not the other way round. However, our attitudes can cause a disruption in the dynamic organization of these two meridians. Impatience, for example, or a desire to finish a project without taking into account the work necessary to realize it, over time can prompt either confusion or competition between the Stomach currents and those of the Spleen-Pancreas. To support the dynamic organization of these meridian lines and better position their pathway through the body, the following protocol can be used.

Sequential Nutripuncture Protocol

For both men and women: 09, 19, 26, 10, 30

Meridian Line 10 of Action

This meridian line provides the necessary information for the Stomach to regulate its activities. It also manages the dynamics of an individual's action, which are normally guided by personal tastes—the desire to move into action, to get excited, to work, to change—in short, their taste for life.

When an action is performed under constraint, without considering the available possibilities and one's own limitations, this can induce disturbances of the Stomach meridian line to such an extent that it will sever its connection to the vital currents' network. The following protocol is very helpful for hyperactive individuals, restoring their taste for action and awareness of their own limitations.

Sequential Nutripuncture Protocol

For women: 10, 27, 33, 30, 16 + 26, 10, 33, 08, 35

For men: 10, 27, 33, 30, 16 + 26, 10, 33, 08, 36

Meridian Line 18 of Transformation

Because of the information it is responsible for circulating, this meridian line ensures the balance of Spleen and Pancreas. It governs the capacity for realization, resulting from the concrete action of the Stomach. Its circulation is closely related to that of meridian line 10 because when we do not manage to move into action, this meridian line will not be able to concretely manifest our capacities for transformation.

Sequential Nutripuncture Protocol

For women: 30, 18, 33, 37, 34 + 18, 33, 26, 08, 12

For men: 30, 18, 33, 38, 34 + 18, 33, 26, 08, 12

Meridian Lines 28 and 21 of Anchoring and Realization

The peak of life's pleasures materializes in men through the creation of life (projection of life) and in the woman by childbirth (manifestation of life). Any deviation of meridian lines 21 or 28 can create a favorable terrain for disorders affecting the Prostate or Uterus. In the event of infertility, it is important to activate these circuits individually to restore these meridian lines to their full potential.

Sequential Nutripuncture Protocol

For women: 28, 33, 01, 29, 37 + 28, 26, 33, 12, 02

For men: 21, 33, 01, 29, 38 + 21, 26, 33, 12, 02

Relieving the Congestion of the Pelvic Region

In the event of pelvic congestion or heaviness, which can often be responsible for painful periods, a meridian called Tchong Mai or the "Marvelous Meridian" can be regulated. It has a very distinctive pathway that wends its way horizontally around the waist, like a belt. Its harmonious circulation relieves congestion of both the Uterus and Prostate.

Sequential Nutripuncture Protocol

For women: 28, 09, 22, 29, 15

For men: 21, 09, 22, 29, 15

Meridian Line 17 of Structuring

The vital currents of structuring ensure proper skeletal density. They regulate gravitational pressures, an essential task for the balance of the body's skeleton. On the mental level, too, the currents of meridian line 17 make it possible for us to "keep our feet on the ground." In situations when we feel like we're falling apart, it is often because the stress of life has weakened these vital currents responsible for securing our verticality and composure for confronting outside events.

Sequential Nutripuncture Protocol

For women: 35, 15, 17, 11, 30 + 02, 34, 26, 17, 27

For men: 36, 15, 17, 11, 30 + 02, 34, 26, 17, 27

Meridian Line 26 of Motor Control

The action of this meridian, governed by the Stomach/Spleen-Pancreas family, involves all the motor systems at the cerebral level: the thalamus and gray matter are the meeting point of these various circuits. For overactive persons who have based their life on their skills and never have given anything away for nothing, this meridian line can affect the cerebral dynamic, weakening the motor system that governs the guidance of action. One can then use the following Sequential Nutripuncture protocol.

Sequential Nutripuncture Protocol

For women: 26, 37, 33, 10, 30 + 26, 12, 31, 34, 28

For men: 26, 38, 33, 10, 30 + 26, 12, 31, 34, 21

The Gustatory Function: The Mouth and the Uterus, the Mouth and the Prostate

Nutripuncture research has shown that sensory perception operates on two levels: one is cerebral (neural integration), and the other is hormonal (emotional construction, the result of the visceral reactions spawned by our sensations). Evidence has thus been provided to demonstrate that our five senses have extremely fine "corporeal interlocutors" and "sexual antenna" capable of decoding the emotional nature of a sensory impression, which is often inaccessible mentally. The important point is to recognize two streams of information. One stream is the visceral

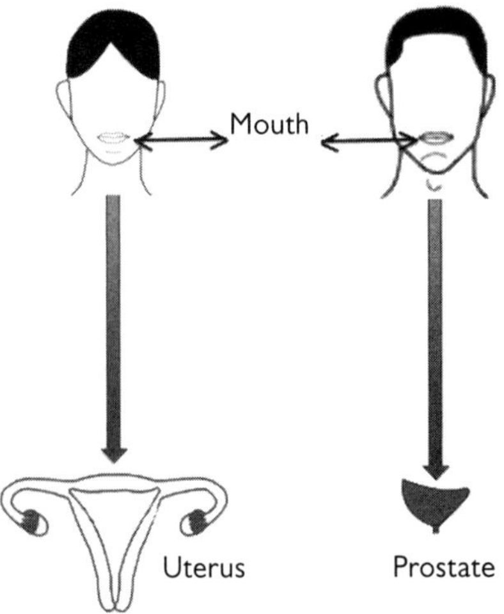

Fig. 14.1. The Mouth is connected to the Uterus in women and the Prostate in men via meridian lines 28 and 21.

brain, which provides the sensory input of basic and instinctual perception deriving from sensation. The second stream is in relationship to the cognitive brain that integrates the information of the five senses. The organism lives with these two streams, which are balanced by the cerebral cortex. Difficulties arise when the cerebral cortex cannot balance these two interdependent streams.

In fact, each sensory receptor located at the cerebral level has its correspondent in the biological terrain, which is to say in the pelvis in regard to the sexual pole. This is why in respect to taste, our mouth is connected to the Uterus, if we are women, or to the Prostate, if we are men, via meridian lines 28 and 21 (fig. 14.1). When these meridian lines are invigorated using a simple Associative Nutripuncture protocol of Nutri Yin–Nutri Yang followed by Nutri 28 or 21, we can restore to our taste all its sensitivity and vitality.

Refining our taste allows us to find a better fit with our lives and regain our footing when we lack an anchor. This makes it possible to find solid roots and the composure necessary for building a solid life. Disturbance of this sense can degenerate into food disorders such as anorexia or bulimia. The common denominator of these disorders is often a rejection of one's body, hence the value of Sequential Nutripuncture, which helps us to accept our body just the way it is. To refine our taste and restore it to its proper place in our overall sensory perception, the following protocol is suggested.

Sequential Nutripuncture Protocol

For women: 28, 33, 27, 15, 26 + 02, 08, 12, 03, 26

For men: 21, 33, 27, 15, 26 + 02, 08, 12, 03, 26

THE KIDNEYS/BLADDER FAMILY

Reminder: This family governs the sense of hearing and relates to the element Water. It presides over the formation of urogenital equipment and the sexual organs in accordance with the chromosomal identity XX or XY. It also adjusts the genetic information we inherit and ensures the integrity of the family lineage.

The Kidneys/Bladder pair also governs memory, whether genetic or acquired. While these meridian lines connect us with our original cellular memory, they also convey information concerning the end of our existence: the death of the body and its cells. Birth and death evoke the cycle of life as it pertains to our family dynamic. The recognition of our origins is thus as important as that of death; it is an inescapable phase of life.

In the circadian cycle, the meridian line of the Bladder is more active between 3 p.m. and 5 p.m. Then, the circulation of the Kidneys meridian line takes over between 5 p.m. and 7 p.m. The Bladder meridian line therefore pours its energy back into the Kidney meridian line. On the mental level, it is alertness and lucidity that brings confidence and self-assurance, not vice versa. Sometimes our behavioral attitudes can affect the natural sequencing of these meridians.

To strengthen the dynamic organization of these meridians and better position their pathways through the body, we can regulate the following circuit.

Sequential Nutripuncture Protocol

For both men and women: 05, 31, 37, 13, 22

Meridian Line 31 of Alertness

With its sixty-seven points, located on parallel branches on either side of the spine, this line constitutes, on the one hand, a mirror of every organ (through its points known as "approvals") and, on the other hand, it assumes the specific role of circulating the necessary information for the Bladder's self-regulation.

When the Bladder exhibits a functional disorder without any obvious cause, it is because an imbalance exists within this meridian line, often induced by a psychosomatic stress. Sometimes a lack of clarity or vigilance, or a refusal to face reality, is the reflection of poor circulation in this meridian line. Here the individual is only fooling himself, pulling the wool over his own eyes and living in complete illusion, thinking the moon is really "made of green cheese." To invigorate meridian line 31 and get more clarity and alertness, the following protocol is useful.

Sequential Nutripuncture Protocol

For women: 09, 33, 29, 27, 31 + 22, 12, 31, 02, 30

For men: 09, 33, 29, 27, 31 + 22, 12, 31, 02, 30

The Bladder muscle also plays a fundamental role in the body's posture, like a tensor of the muscular system in relation to the different fascia (aponeuroses connecting the different muscle chains). If this muscle is flaccid and lacks tone, the following meridian lines can be stimulated.

Sequential Nutripuncture Protocol

For women: 23, 31, 16, 05, 33 + 24, 23, 16, 34, 08

For men: 23, 31, 16, 05, 33 + 24, 23, 16, 34, 08

Meridian Line 22 of Assurance

In apprehensive, introverted, or shy people, this meridian line is always disturbed. To regain self-confidence and to outgrow certain fears, the connections in this network of vital currents can be reinforced.

Sequential Nutripuncture Protocol

For women: 22, 33, 11, 30, 37 + 29, 08, 22, 23, 02

For men: 22, 33, 11, 30, 38 + 29, 08, 22, 23, 02

Meridian Line 09 of the Source

This meridian line, in relation to the metabolism of water, controls the circulation of our ancestral vitality. This is the reason it is called the "meridian of the source." If an individual is experiencing a chronic lack of mental or physical vitality, its connections in the meridian network can be stimulated to awaken his or her vital potential.

Sequential Nutripuncture Protocol

For women: 22, 31, 01, 29, 15 + 12, 08, 09, 34, 27

For men: 22, 31, 01, 29, 15 + 12, 08, 09, 34, 27

Meridian Line 29 of Receptivity

The dynamic of this meridian line, already mentioned above, ensures venous receptivity as well as the ability to receive in general. To stimulate this dynamic the following circuits can be regulated.

Sequential Nutripuncture Protocol

For women: 29, 09, 33, 35, 23 + 30, 15, 35, 29, 08

For men: 29, 09, 33, 36, 23 + 30, 15, 36, 29, 08

Meridian Lines 09 and 29: The Dynamic of the Gonads

The interaction of meridians 09 and 29 feeds the vitality of the Gonads (Ovaries and Testicles), which are involved in the hormonal and thus the emotional dynamic of the individual. While they can be jointly stimulated with a simple Associative Nutripuncture protocol of Nutri Yin–Nutri Yang followed by Nutri 09 + Nutri 29, sometimes a specific Sequential Nutripuncture protocol is recommended to provide a profound adjustment to hormonal balance. Among adolescents, for example, this specific protocol makes it possible to improve skin condition (such as acne) and to regulate the menstrual cycle. It also permits shy people to communicate more easily, without fear.

Nutripuncture research has made it possible to confirm the existence of an informational relationship between the Gonads and auditory functions. In fact, by stimulating the meridians involved in the balance of the Gonads, improved hearing has been observed, as well as an ability to tune in more deeply to oneself and others.

Sequential Nutripuncture Protocol

For women: 29, 09, 37, 33, 11 + 29, 23, 02, 34, 08

For men: 29, 09, 38, 33, 11 + 29, 23, 02, 34, 08

Meridian Line 27 of Time

Reminder: This meridian line controls our biorhythms and our ability to anchor in space and time, indispensable for spatial orientation (meridian lines 28 for women, and 21 for men). This meridian line is involved in the rhythmic sequence of many bodily functions, thereby supporting self-regulation of the body's biorhythms. Various biological or psychological disorders can arise from an imbalance of this meridian line. Whether circulation is reduced or excessive, it is important to help it assume its crucial role and position in the network of all the vital currents.

In the event of jet lag, especially in particularly sensitive people, one can use a specific Sequential Nutripuncture that respectively stimulates the meridians as follows.

Sequential Nutripuncture Protocol

For women: 31, 09, 27, 35, 32 + 27, 31, 02, 12, 08

For men: 31, 09, 27, 36, 32 + 27, 31, 02, 12, 08

Meridian Line 23 of Representation

Each part of the eye is connected with specific meridian lines; the Kidneys/Bladder pair governs the balance of retinal function. The sensation of eyestrain is not necessarily connected to the retina itself but to the information that is possibly interfering with its function. If Associative Nutripuncture is not sufficient to reduce potential eyestrain (with the use of Nutri Yin–Nutri Yang and Nutris 23 and 32), a Sequential Nutripuncture protocol can be used to invigorate these circuits.

Sequential Nutripuncture Protocol

For women: 23, 08, 11, 32, 37 + 24, 03, 02, 32, 01

For men: 23, 08, 11, 32, 38 + 24, 03, 02, 32, 01

Meridian Line 02 of Postural Balance

This meridian line, in synergy with meridian line 31, ensures the balance of biped posture. In the event of dizziness, there is often a destabilization caused by psychological interferences: fear, overwork, side effects from other stresses, and so forth. The following sequence will put meridian line 02 back in tune with the overall dynamic of the body.

Sequential Nutripuncture Protocol

For women: 09, 31, 34, 29, 23 + 31, 09, 26, 02, 11

For men: 09, 31, 34, 29, 23 + 31, 09, 26, 02, 11

For the practitioner though, it is always helpful to seek out the cause of a vital current's deviation. For example, each time a disturbance of meridian line 02 (Cerebellum) is connected with meridians 04 (Heart) and 30 (Gall Bladder), it probably indicates a latent Oedipal problem (see chapter 11), which can come to the surface at the time of a profound emotional stress connected with a relationship.

The Auditory Function: The Ears and the Gonads

As we saw earlier concerning the gustatory function, we have extremely fine "corporeal interlocutors" and "sexual antenna" capable of decoding the emotional nature of a sensory impression. With respect to the Ears, they are related to the Gonads (Ovaries or Testicles) via meridian lines 29 and 09 (fig. 14.2). This is why when these meridians are stimulated with a simple Associative Nutripuncture protocol of Nutri Yin–Nutri Yang plus Nutris 09 and 29, our ability to hear and listen will be deeper, making it possible for us to globally evaluate resonance of the sound vibrations, using our entire body.

All hearing deficiencies are related to a profound disruption of the Kidneys/Bladder family, in particular its secondary meridians related to the Gonads. In the event of hearing loss, it is therefore a good idea to also adjust the vital currents of the Gonads. The expression "to be all ears," evokes the receptivity that is essential for producing sound: without hearing there is no access to verbal language. Hearing, like the voice, should be properly positioned and fit well at a point between the upper and lower halves of the body, in order to ensure optimal reception. This is accomplished by stimulating the following meridian lines.

Sequential Nutripuncture Protocol

For women: 22, 02, 09, 15, 24 + 03, 09, 29, 02, 08

For men: 22, 02, 09, 15, 14 + 03, 09, 29, 02, 08

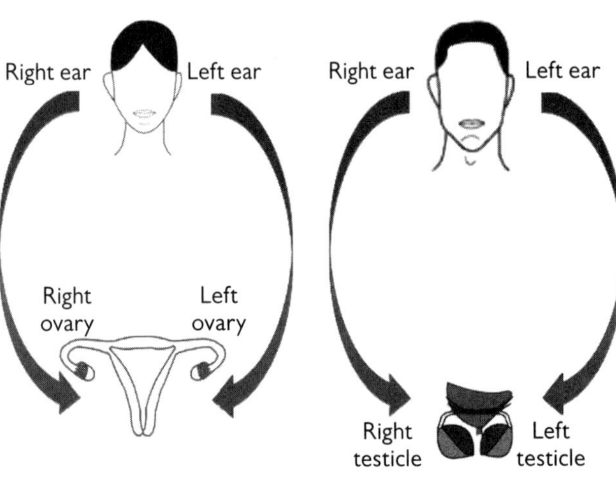

Fig. 14.2. The Ears are related to the Gonads via meridian lines 29 and 09.

Vocalization

Vocalization calls upon several structures: the jaws, the vocal cords, the tongue, the palate, the lungs, It is also not foreign to hormonal activity and gender expression. In fact, the tone of the voice is one of the sexual characteristics that change at puberty.

Hearing and vocalization are two closely linked functions: one permits the flowering of the other. While the first is receptive, the latter is a projection of sound. These functions mutually nourish each other. This is the reason why for tuning one's voice, we also use a protocol to invigorate hearing. Once the auditory instrument has been thoroughly awakened, the voice will naturally set or tune itself without any effort. To tune your voice, for us, means to anchor it within your lower body, which will enable it to act as an instrument of resonance. To enable the voice "to take root" the following sequence is recommended.

Sequential Nutripuncture Protocol

For women: 35, 25, 29, 09, 24 + 23, 09, 24, 37, 08

For men: 35, 25, 29, 09, 14 + 23, 09, 14, 38, 08

THE LUNGS/COLON FAMILY

This family brings an individual flavor to our action, polarizing it in accordance with our gender. The sense of smell, governed by the element Air, is master and governs individual feelings.

In the circadian cycle, the meridian line of the Lung is more active between 3 a.m. and 5 a.m. Then the circulation of the meridian line of the Colon takes over and becomes more constant between 5 a.m. and 7 a.m. It is therefore the energy of the Lung meridian line that pours back into that of the Colon and not vice versa. On a symbolic level, when you have found your inspiration, your breath (Lungs), you can organize yourself (Colon) based on your polarity (gender).

Sometimes our habitual behaviors can induce disturbances to this sequence and prepare a favorable terrain for certain respiratory disorders. In asthma, for example, we often find a psychosomatic component representing an inversion of the dynamic organization of these meridian lines. To reinforce the synergy of these vital currents and better position their pathway through the body, the following sequence is recommended.

Sequential Nutripuncture Protocol

For both men and women: 20, 33, 30, 34, 05

Meridian Line 20 of Breath

This meridian line governs vitality of the respiratory function and ensures self-regulation of the lungs. When air enters the respiratory tract, it is analyzed and recognized by the olfactory system. Then the information present in the ambient air is normally adopted, or integrated on the cerebral level by the rhinencephalon (which captures and memorizes olfactory intake). When pollens present in the air are not recognized, they can cause reactions such as a sinus infection. In any allergic reactions, the balance of meridian line 20 is always weakened, as well as meridian lines 25 and 12.

There is also a very close relationship between the Kidneys/Bladder family, which manages the genetic legacy (origin) and the Lungs/Colon family, which makes it possible to give an individual flavor to this legacy. With this relationship in mind, it is important to reinforce the recognition of our origin (evoking the analogy between pollens, vegetable gametes, and the gametes from which we came) and the adoption of our body. This makes it possible to strengthen the biological terrain upon which respiratory disorders can develop, disorders which are sometimes of an allergic nature. Therefore, to restore vitality to meridian line 20 and reinforce its dynamic in the vital current network, the following protocol is recommended.

Sequential Nutripuncture Protocol

For women: 29, 01, 11, 15, 20 + 32, 37, 20, 25, 12

For men: 29, 01, 11, 15, 20 + 32, 38, 20, 25, 12

Respiratory Balance and the Body Diagram

The respiratory dynamic can be disturbed at times by an erroneous spatial representation of the right and left Lung. Due to its symmetrical course, meridian line 20 feeds these two functionally similar but anatomically different organs (two lobes on the left lung and three lobes on the right lung). Following an emotional shock, the symmetrical circulation of this meridian line can be reversed, distorting the body diagram, and thereby disrupting the respiratory dynamic. To correct the symmetrical spatial representation of meridian line 20, the following sequence is recommended.

Sequential Nutripuncture Protocol

For women: 35, 20, 33, 30, 37
For men: 36, 20, 33, 30, 38

Meridian Line 05 of Organization

The role of this meridian line, complementary to the meridian line of the Lungs, ensures the balance of gaseous exchanges and intestinal peristalsis. The organ to which it is connected, the Colon, is very sensitive to hormonal fluctuations and also has a great influence on sexual expression. Its rhythm, influenced by the information of its neural plexuses (Auerbach's plexus and Meissner's plexus), is very sensitive to the environment and related lifestyle changes. The Colon meridian line modulates the individual's "organizational" faculties and the ability to prioritize tasks. If you want to restore the Colon's vitality within the organism's overall balance, the following sequence is recommended.

Sequential Nutripuncture Protocol

For women: 16, 09, 15, 05, 12 + 05, 12, 24, 02, 11
For men: 16, 09, 15, 05, 12 + 05, 12, 14, 02, 11

Meridian Line 25 of Inspiration

This meridian line controls the recognition of aromatic information, plays an active role in balancing air cavities, olfactory perception, and the expression of feeling. Its dynamics are closely related to that of meridian line 12, regulating the balance of the rhinencephalon. This vital current can be activated in a very simple way by using the Associative Nutripuncture protocol of Nutri Yin–Nutri Yang plus Nutris 25 and 12, but to restore its full vitality and put it back in step with the overall circulation of its network, the following sequence is recommended.

Sequential Nutripuncture Protocol

For women: 24, 12, 07, 25, 15 + 25, 37, 15, 12, 08
For men: 14, 12, 06, 25, 15 + 25, 38, 15, 12, 08

Meridian Line 12 of Instinct

This meridian provides support to the rhinencephalon, which collects the olfactory impulses in synergy with meridian line 25. It is very sensitive to stress and overwork—both physical and mental—and plays a very important role in hormonal balance. In the event of overwork, it is very helpful to support and reinforce its connections in the general network of the vital currents with the following sequence.

Sequential Nutripuncture Protocol

For women: 15, 35, 34, 20, 32 + 37, 34, 15, 12, 31

For men: 15, 36, 34, 20, 32 + 38, 34, 15, 12, 31

Meridian Line 16 of Movement

This meridian relates to the movement fueled by breathing, a movement essential to life. Its dynamic is therefore closely tied to that of meridian line 20. Flexibility on the psychophysical level is the fundamental characteristic these meridians provide. When a loss of elasticity or an overly dogmatic attitude is in evidence, the vitality of meridian line 16 can be sustained with a specific protocol that strengthens its connection with the vital current network.

Sequential Nutripuncture Protocol

For women: 16, 37, 31, 18, 30 + 16, 08, 33, 26, 02

For men: 16, 38, 31, 18, 30 + 16, 08, 33, 26, 02

Meridian Line 15 of Self-Expression

This meridian line plays a fundamental role in the dynamic of tissue recognition. The information it carries supports our immunity. Stimulating it offers support to the vitality of the immune system.

Sequential Nutripuncture Protocol

For women: 25, 15, 33, 24, 07 + 25, 05, 15, 12, 13

For men: 25, 15, 33, 14, 06 + 25, 05, 15, 12, 13

Meridian Line 24 of Femininity

Meridian line 24 is activated at the time of puberty to express the female sensitivity of the young woman. The activation of this meridian line—harmonious or not—depends on individual experience and the context in which this transition unfolded, and the depth of the desire to express one's femininity. Once adulthood is reached, diet, hormonal secretions, sexual activity, and social relations are some of the many elements capable of compromising the balance of these vital currents. If a woman is seeking to express all the power of her femininity, the following two sequences are recommended.

Sequential Nutripuncture Protocol

29, 15, 27, 24, 09, followed by 24, 33, 04, 08, 32

Meridian Line 14 of Virility

This meridian line is activated by puberty, when the larynx of the young boy changes under the hormonal impregnation: the voice changes and acquires a deeper tone. Through his voice, the young man thus starts to affirm his virility, marking his entrance to adult life. When a man has trouble asserting himself or expressing his virility though his voice, he can stimulate the following meridian lines.

Sequential Nutripuncture Protocol

36, 01, 04, 15, 14, followed by 01, 32, 14, 08, 38

Meridian Line 07 of Female Sexuality

With puberty, hormonal secretions prompt the activation of this secondary meridian line, which plays a role in female sexual communication. It is introspective and complementary to the more projective male sexual expression, animated by meridian line 06. In order to improve the expression of her female polarity and her relations with the opposite sex, a woman can stimulate meridians using the following sequences.

Sequential Nutripuncture Protocol

25, 15, 33, 37, 07, followed by 05, 12, 07, 08, 33

Meridian Line 06 of Male Sexuality

Hormonal secretions during puberty trigger the activation of this secondary meridian line, which modulates male sexual communication. It is projective and complementary to the more introspective female sexual expression, animated by meridian line 07. In order to improve the expression of their male polarity and their relations with the opposite sex, men should invigorate the following sequence of meridians.

Sequential Nutripuncture Protocol

25, 15, 33, 38, 06, followed by 05, 12, 06, 08, 33

The Olfactory Function: The Nose and the Vagina, the Nose and the Penis

The corporeal interlocutor for the sense of smell finds its corresponding agent in the pelvis for the nose in either the Vagina (women) or the Penis (men). Invigorating these meridian lines, in combination with meridian line 25, makes it possible for the olfactory faculty to recover its full sensitivity, while awakening its feeling. Scent has always been synonymous with being "clued in" and getting the picture, as shown by such expressions as "smell a rat," or something doesn't "smell right." Getting in step with your sense of smell is essential for expressing your male or female individuality, and for finding inspiration. A reduced sense of smell makes a favorable terrain for various disorders to appear, especially those of an allergic nature. Disruptions of the sense of smell are a precursory sign of certain neurological diseases such as Parkinson's.

Every individual has a distinct odor, the result of his or her metabolism, which is as much a sign of individual identity as fingerprints or DNA code. Body odor is an emanation, an essence given off by the cellular labor involved in metabolic transformation. It is therefore the process of action and change that generates odors.

To refine our smell proves to be an essential action for allowing the information under our olfactory perception's control to flow. Indeed, odorous information acting on sexual hormonal secretions plays a fundamental part in psychophysical balance. One can therefore stimulate the following circuits.

Sequential Nutripuncture Protocol

For women: 07, 35, 25, 33, 22 + 03, 12, 25, 08, 15
For men: 06, 36, 25, 33, 22 + 03, 12, 25, 08, 15

THE HEART/SMALL INTESTINE FAMILY

Reminder: This family is connected with the element Fire and governs vision, in particular the anterior chamber of the eye, allowing the projection of the gaze—in other words, the power to see. This pair is connected with the Cerebral Cortex, the outermost layer of the highly developed human brain.

In the circadian cycle, the meridian line of the Heart is more active between 11 a.m. and 1 p.m. Then, the circulation of the meridian line of the Small Intestine takes over and becomes more constant between 1 p.m. and 3 p.m. It is therefore the energy of the meridian line of the Heart that animates the meridian line of the Small Intestine and not the other way around. By following your intuition and the way you choose to look at things (Heart), you can make better choices (Small Intestine).

Sometimes our attitude can disrupt this sequence and prepare a favorable terrain for some ocular visual sphere disorders as well as for problems affecting assimilation. For example, when you make a choice guided by fear rather than your true desire and personal plans for your life, you disrupt the dynamic of this pair of meridians. To strengthen the dynamic organization of these vital currents and improve their pathway's position in the body, the following sequence is recommended.

Sequential Nutripuncture Protocol

For both men and women: 04, 22, 13, 11, 31

Meridian Line 08 of Cognitive Integration

The Cerebral Cortex forms the command center of the organism. This is why it is recommended that its meridian line be stimulated on a regular basis. The management of the vast amount of information with which it needs to deal and integrate can overwork the Cerebral Cortex. It can be strengthened in a very simple way with an Associative Nutripuncture protocol of Nutri Yin–Nutri Yang plus Nutri 08. Several other factors can affect the balance of the Cerebral Cortex. One of these is the metabolic center, its complementary pole. The regulation of its meridian lines, 11 and 30 conjointly with meridian line 06, is always helpful. A spatio-temporal imbalance can also disrupt its performance. If this is the case, the vital currents of spatio-temporal anchoring (27 and 28 for women, 27 and 21 for men), in combination with meridian line 08, can be stimulated.

If you wish to restore the full dynamic of meridian line 08, the following circuits can be activated.

Sequential Nutripuncture Protocol

For women: 03, 34, 08, 32, 35 + 20, 16, 04, 30, 37

For men: 03, 34, 08, 32, 36 + 20, 16, 04, 30, 38

Meridian Line 04 of Decision and Rhythm

Heart rhythm depends on various regulating cores (Keith–Flack node, node of Aschoff and Tawara, bundle of His), animated by circuits of particular meridian lines. Other rhythmic systems can condition its dynamic, in particular those relating to the Colon (Meissner and Auerbach). There are many factors capable of interfering with the balance of its meridian line.

Emotional stress can affect its circulation and weaken the biological terrain of the organ to which it is connected. For this reason, following a stress of a sentimental nature, it is important to stimulate the potential of this meridian line in order to better manage our emotions. In this case, we reinforce its connections in the general network of the following vital currents.

Sequential Nutripuncture Protocol

For women: 04, 01, 32, 08, 34 + 32, 08, 04, 02, 26

For men: 04, 01, 32, 08, 34 + 32, 08, 04, 02, 26

Meridian Line 13 of Choice

These currents feed an organ that consists of three parts performing different functions: duodenum, jejunum, and ileum. The Small Intestine plays a fundamental role in immunity (lymphocytes) and in the re-absorption process. Its balance is related to the information it has, via its meridian line, to recognize all ingested foods. Thus, when the circulation of meridian line 13 is disturbed, the Small Intestine does not manage to recognize certain foods any longer. Some forms of food intolerance (lactose, casein, gluten) can then appear.

Regulating these vital currents encourages optimal re-absorption. On the psychological level, the threefold nature of digestive capacity is demonstrated in the ability to choose guided by preconceived plans (Heart).

Sequential Nutripuncture Protocol

For women: 13, 37, 20, 33, 15 + 13, 32, 08, 15, 37

For men: 13, 38, 20, 33, 15 + 13, 32, 08, 15, 38

Meridian Line 01 of the Gift

This meridian line controls blood circulation, in particular the impulse and the projection of blood in the arteries. This impulse, which is both physical and mental, takes place in synergy with the venous return, allowing the exchange and sharing of resources. On the behavioral level, this circulation is seen in our ability to approach others, by the capacity to give (artery) but also to receive (veins). To refine and sharpen these communicational abilities, we can support the system of arterial communication with the following sequences.

Sequential Nutripuncture Protocol

For women: 01, 34, 04, 08, 32 + 37, 11, 01, 08, 02

For men: 01, 34, 04, 08, 32 + 38, 11, 01, 08, 02

Meridian Line 32 of Sight

This meridian line controls the anterior chamber of the Eye in its role as projector of the gaze. It enables us to clarify reality according to our individual mental projections. On the other hand, its complementary meridian line 23 ensures our visual reception, related to the posterior chamber of the eye. A simple Associative Nutripuncture protocol of Nutri Yin–Nutri Yang plus Nutris 23 and 32 is sufficient to activate this meridian line, in combination with its complementary meridians, and ensure a better visual acuity.

The Visual Function: Look and You Shall See!

Our outlook plays a key role in the expression of our humanity. Our visual impressions depend on the outlook we have on reality, often conditioned by our cellular memory, resulting from past experiences. Each structure of the eye is combined with specific meridian lines in connection with the five families. Their balance or imbalance can therefore have a direct impact upon our visual function.

Projecting our own outlook, the mirror of our cognitive identity, is a fundamental action that makes it possible for us to fully express all our vitality. This is expressed at the level of the sexual pole through the clitoris and the cervix for women, and the glans for men, which are both animated by the same vital currents. In order to restore a proper outlook that harmonizes with your true self, you can use the following protocol.

Sequential Nutripuncture Protocol

For women: 32, 37, 23, 33, 08 + 12, 08, 32, 37, 34
For men: 32, 38, 23, 33, 08 + 12, 08, 32, 38, 34

Vision and Restorative Sleep

Some of us have trouble getting restful sleep because of a disturbance in the cerebral systems, subjacent to the Cerebral Cortex. To invigorate the circuits of the meridian lines involved in this imbalance makes it possible to benefit from the rejuvenating effects of a restful sleep.

Sequential Nutripuncture Protocol

For women: 22, 09, 02, 11, 32 + 03, 19, 23, 02, 11
For men: 22, 09, 02, 11, 32 + 03, 19, 23, 02, 11

THE LIVER/GALL BLADDER FAMILY, HALF OF THE DOUBLE FAMILY OF MERIDIANS

Reminder: As the metabolic blood pole, this family activates and regulates energy flow. Its activity complements that of the cerebral neural pole. The synergy of these two poles governs the sense of touch, related to the element Boundary (Ether) and ensures the vitality and proper placement of each organ.

In the circadian cycle, the meridian line of the Gall Bladder is more active between 11 p.m and 1 a.m. Then the circulation of the meridian line of the Liver takes over and becomes more constant between 1 and 3 in the morning. It is therefore the energy of the Gall Bladder that pours back into the Liver currents and not vice versa. Sometimes our attitudes can induce disruptions to this sequence and prepare a terrain that will be favorable for the creation of certain digestive and behavioral disorders. To reinforce the dynamic organization of these meridian lines and better position their pathway through the body, the following sequence is recommended.

Sequential Nutripuncture Protocol

For women: 30, 11, 33, 37, 09

For men: 30, 11, 33, 38, 09

Meridian Line 11 of Metabolic Activation

A heavy demand is placed in these circuits, as they play a major role in activating the body's energy center: the Liver. When a person's body is severely overworked (too much food, alcohol, physical labor), it is under great strain and this condition can induce irritating and aggressive attitudes, often spontaneous and difficult to be controlled by the cerebral pole. In this case, it is important to strengthen the connections of this meridian line in the general network of vital currents in the following sequence.

Sequential Nutripuncture Protocol

For women: 37, 29, 11, 33, 13 + 33, 35, 11, 08, 12

For men: 38, 29, 11, 33, 13 + 33, 36, 11, 08, 12

Meridian Line 30 of Metabolic Regulation

Meridian line 30, the partner of meridian line 11, plays a major role in metabolic regulation, purification of blood, emulsion of fat, the draining of excess bodily fluids, and so on. This meridian line is always disturbed in people who are not able "to digest" overwhelming or painful experiences, who contend with feelings of rancor and bitterness. Providing support to its balance, in combination with that of meridian line 11, encourages optimal vitality on both the mental and physical level.

Sequential Nutripuncture Protocol

For women: 18, 30, 35, 13, 04 + 30, 37, 03, 23, 08

For men: 18, 30, 36, 13, 04 + 30, 38, 03, 23, 08

Remove Toxins from Your Blood—and Starve Mosquitoes!

People whose meridians 11 and 30 are overburdened and overworked will feel chronically exhausted and generally somnolent. This is due to the metabolic pole's inability to ensure the cleansing of the body. Two specific circuits of meridians can be called upon in this case to prompt the elimination of the toxins in the blood that are responsible for this discomfort.

Thanks to live observation of the figurative elements in blood (white and red corpuscles and so on), with the help of a special microscope, several Italian practitioners have observed that an individual's blood (sometimes very thick and dense) would become much more fluid after using the following protocol. The people who have tried this have noticed that it also made them less prone to getting bitten by mosquitoes.

Sequential Nutripuncture Protocol

For women: 35, 01, 11, 37, 30 + 30, 26, 37, 34, 08

For men: 36, 01, 11, 38, 30 + 30, 26, 38, 34, 08

THE MASTER OF THE HEART/TRIPLE WARMER FAMILY, HALF OF THE DOUBLE FAMILY OF MERIDIANS

Reminder: These meridian lines are regulators of the organism. They modulate and contain the metabolic impulse of the Liver/Gall Bladder family. The information conveyed by the 35/36 and 37/38 pairs ensures neuro-sensory balance and controls excesses in the event of hypo- or hyper–neuro-vegetative excitability.

In the circadian cycle, the meridian line of the Master of Heart is more active between 7 p.m. and 9 p.m. Then the circulation of the Triple Heater meridian line takes the relay and becomes more constant between 9 p.m. and 11 p.m. It is therefore the energy of the master of the Heart that flows into the Triple Warmer and not the other way round. Our behavior can cause disturbances in the smooth functioning of this sequence and prepare a favorable terrain for the appearance of some skin problems and nervous disorders. To reinforce the dynamic organization of these vital currents and better place their pathways through our body, the following circuit can be regulated.

Sequential Nutripuncture Protocol

For women: 35, 27, 09, 02, 37

For men: 36, 27, 09, 02, 38

We can compare these meridian lines to an electrician (Master of the Heart) and a heating specialist (Triple Warmer). They ensure the settings and boundaries of each organ and polarize all the body's sectors according to the sexual characteristics of the individual. In synergy with the metabolic pole, they support cerebral balance, as well as the balance of the skin and mucous membranes (the sense of touch). In synergy with the 33/34 pair, they govern spatial organization.

Meridian Lines 35 and 36 of Neural Activation

To support the balance of meridians 35/36, we can invigorate their connections in the network of the vital currents.

Sequential Nutripuncture Protocol

For women: 04, 32, 35, 33, 02 + 29, 02, 01, 35, 33

For men: 04, 32, 36, 33, 02 + 29, 02, 01, 36, 33

Meridian Lines 37 and 38 of Neural Regulation

To support the balance of meridians 37/38 we can stimulate their connections in the network of the vital currents.

Sequential Nutripuncture Protocol

For women: 33, 11, 13, 37, 02 + 12, 02, 26, 19, 27

For men: 33, 11, 13, 38, 02 + 12, 02, 26, 19, 27

Tactile Function: Hair and the Perineum

Skin, headquarters for the sense of touch, ensures, on the one hand, the layout of the body and, on the other hand, it forms an interactive surface between the inside and outside. The tactile field is a very elaborate system of recognition that only humans have developed to this degree. It makes intimate contact possible thanks to the exchange of large amounts of information. This makes possible a profound form of communication that spoken language often finds impossible to duplicate. Hair and the perineum (the vulva for women and the scrotum for men) are particularly sensitive, which gives them a starring role in the domain of touch.

While all the meridian lines take part indirectly in the balance of touch, the two poles that regulate the body play a major role in its neural and metabolic dynamic. To sustain the balance of the tactile function, these same circuits can be stimulated for maintaining skin balance.

Sequential Nutripuncture Protocol

For women: 19, 27, 03, 08, 33 + 19, 32, 08, 33, 34

For men: 19, 27, 03, 08, 33 + 19, 32, 08, 33, 34

Meridian Line 19 of Contact

The vital currents of the skin manage the body's boundaries and its "fit" in space. On the mental level, these currents regulate the ability to establish contact. Some kinds of psychophysical stress can weaken their circulation and adversely affect the individual's integrity. To support the vitality of this meridian line as well as its connections in the vital current network, a specific protocol can be used.

Sequential Nutripuncture Protocol

For women: 19, 27, 03, 08, 33 + 19, 32, 03, 33, 34

For men: 19, 27, 03, 08, 33 + 19, 32, 03, 33, 34

Meridian Line 03 of Potency

This meridian adjusts the strength and potency of each individual in reflection of his or her uniqueness. When contact or connection with the self is lost, these vital currents are always affected. Their circulation and connection in the vital current network can be supported with a specific protocol.

Sequential Nutripuncture Protocol

For women: 03, 27, 31, 22, 37 + 03, 08, 01, 32, 02

For men: 03, 27, 31, 22, 38 + 03, 08, 01, 32, 02

Meridian Line 33 of Orientation

Working in synergy with meridian line 34, this meridian manages the energy axis of the body—the central path of human verticality, the connection between the perineum and the mouth—and the ability to orient oneself in space. It allows one to "conceive" of life and engender it. The following protocol will strengthen the vitality of this essential, fundamental meridian.

Sequential Nutripuncture Protocol

For women: 33, 11, 30, 37, 04 + 35, 08, 27, 33, 26

For men: 33, 11, 30, 38, 04 + 36, 08, 27, 33, 26

Meridian Line 34 of Orientation

Working in synergy with meridian line 33, this meridian manages the energy axis of the body—the central path of human verticality, the connection between the perineum and the mouth—and the ability to orient oneself in space. It permits the individual to govern her life, to hold its reins. The following protocol will strengthen the vitality of this essential, fundamental meridian.

Sequential Nutripuncture Protocol

For women: 34, 35, 03, 09, 31 + 03, 04, 08, 32, 35

For men: 34, 36, 03, 09, 31 + 03, 04, 08, 32, 36

Conclusion

THE PURPOSE of Nutripuncture is to restore cellular communication and environment-body-individual interaction to its optimum levels. It is based on the logic of complexity (*complex* means "woven together"). The human organism is a complex system, whose dynamic depends, on the one hand, on the flow of information circulating inside it and, on the other hand, the individual ability to deal with and respond to the information received from the environment.

While physical diseases and mental diseases were once considered to be different, today new horizons have been opened by the understanding of psychosomatics. Currently it is believed that there is an emotional component in all diseases and the development of the illness depends in part upon the individual's psychological dynamic.

PNEI (Psycho-Neuro-Endocrine-Immunology) represents an evolution in our understanding of the psychosomatic nature of human beings and has made it possible to show how the psyche has an impact on the central nervous system,

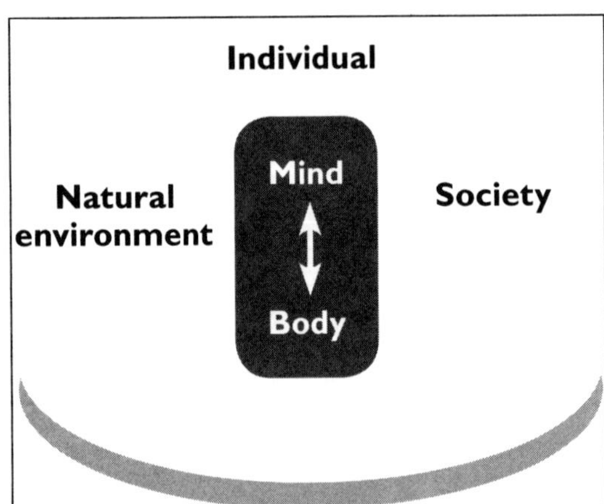

Fig. Concl.1. The purpose of Nutripuncture is to restore cellular communication and environment-body-individual interaction to its optimum levels.

and how this latter interacts with the endocrine and immune systems, thereby determining the development or resolution of the disease. The dynamic of the endocrine and immune systems also interferes with the central nervous system and therefore with the mind (as can be seen in the case of premenstrual irritability or depression).

Another evolution in our understanding of psychosomatics is provided by psycho-epigenetics, which recognizes the mind's ability to interfere with the regulation of DNA, by activating or inhibiting genes. This regulation can also be passed down to following generations. Depending on the epigenetic profile, the mind therefore constitutes an ever-moving milieu that interferes with the evolutionary dynamic of the body. The epigenetic perspective has thus stripped DNA of its role as the cell's "brain" by recognizing it as one element among others that takes part in the permanent dialogue between cells and the environment, the foundation of life's evolutionary dynamic. DNA is therefore like a musical score that the musician (the environment with its stimuli) can play in different ways.

Even on the cellular level, it is rather the phospholipidic membrane, with its proteinaceous receptors, that ensures the dialogue between cell and surroundings and, through an epigenetic process, encourages the activation of genes capable of producing the proteins needed for its dynamic. This process takes place in a complex, organized environment where thousands of chemical reactions are being produced simultaneously.

However, the mystery of life is not found in the biochemical reactions occurring on the cellular level but in the body's incredible capacity to "organize," and its ability to deal with information and respond to it in a consistent manner.

Nutripuncture, through the information provided by its trace element complexes, stimulates the dynamic of the membranes and cellular vitality, ensuring the functional consistency of the various cellular groups. It allows the individual to optimally manage the permanent interaction between body and environment—both human and natural—in order to face sometimes-difficult existential and psychological situations. In this perspective, Nutripuncture provides a very efficient tool, one that can complement all other therapies, for helping the body cope with difficult times and improve the biological terrain in which physical or mental disorders can develop. We continue to move forward in this research to improve individual vitality and the quality of human relationships, a challenge that concerns everyone who cares about building the future of the human community.

The research that began in France in the 1980s at Orsay University has been continued by numerous practitioners (doctors, acupuncturists, osteopaths, psychologists, naturopaths) in different countries (Italy, Belgium, Canada), permitting the perfection of many protocols for maintaining well-being. The thirty-eight trace element complexes developed in 1985 have evolved over time to conform to European Standards. The use of the thirty-eight supplements has made it possible, little by little, to expand our knowledge of human beings and our behavior in response to the events we face in life.

These studies and their application have also made it possible to develop a teaching that tackles the complexity of human behavior and the particular way individuals adjust their vital currents in accordance with their environment. Today, thanks to observation of the permanent interaction between organic life and environment, we have been able to establish connections between different knowledge bases, overcome barriers, and catch sight of a small fraction of the human being's incredible potential.

The knowledge imparted in this book, the result of many years of Nutripuncture research, in itself provides an excellent springboard for "making a fresh start." However, if you wish to discover your body's incredible potential and activate its full vitality, it is necessary to try it for yourself.

To get the best advantage of the information provided in this book and try your own Nutripuncture experience, there are different options available.

- The quickest and simplest way to obtain the benefits offered by this method (when there are no other health priorities) is to stimulate the vital currents based on the seasons, as described in chapter 5.
- We always recommend beginners start with Associative Nutripuncture, an essential "first step" for stimulating physical and mental vitality, and ensuring optimal cellular exchanges, before trying Sequential Nutripuncture. This is detailed in part 2 of the book.
- Next, if you want to explore further and do an in-depth treatment to stimulate a vital potential often inhibited by the stress of living, you can use the Sequential Nutripuncture protocols provided in part 3 of the book.

- However, to draw up a precise and thorough balance sheet that reveals all the defects of your individual biological terrain, its predispositions and behavioral profile, it is a good idea to work with a practitioner who has received training in Nutripuncture.

Please refer to the Resources section (appendix B) for contact information and links to Nutri suppliers, practitioners, workshops, and courses.

APPENDIX A

Nutripuncture, an Ideal Instrument for Supporting Human Communication

ONGOING RESEARCH on gesture and sound communication has made it possible to offer courses on gesture and voice that are open to both professionals and the public at large. In Italy, the Human Voice Association offers training to support the fulfillment of individual cognitive potential, essential for the creation of a human ethic as the base of planetary intercultural communication. More information on the activities of this association can be found at www.human-voice.org.

The goal of this research structure is to cast an overall look at the communication codes of human beings in the light of the interdisciplinary studies that have made it possible to organize the knowledge garnered by Nutripuncture. The work performed by the Human Voice Association offers a way to stimulate individual communication potential—in both gesture and sound—for the purpose of better managing the impact of stress on the quality of human relations.

MOVEMENT, GESTURE, WALKING

Our relational life begins very early in life, as early as intrauterine life when the individual is still a satellite of the "mother planet." Once emerged from this aquatic environment, the baby is propelled into the air, an environment that is rich in stimuli and in which cries and gestures are the first forms of communication, signals that he or she gradually learns to codify. A long breaking-in period, full of pitfalls, awaits all the babies of the world before they become bipedal, talking human beings.

The first movements that prepare posture and walking on two feet have been the subject of a multidisciplinary study[1] seeking to discover their impact on neurological organization, corporeal awakening, motor coordination, and the circulation of the vital currents. Twelve of these so-called archetypal movements have been programmed into our genes and constitute the initial codes, the evolutionary stages of the human gesture repertoire.

Categorized in the 1950s by an American neurosurgeon, Dr. Temple Fay, these spontaneous body movements are practiced from the time of birth by all babies in the world (no matter their race or culture) in order to build vertical posture, learn how to walk on two feet, and organize their neurological networks of intentional movements. The brain, immature at birth, builds its connections thanks to these initial movements of the body. These reflex movements of the baby prepare the dialogue between brain and body by calling upon biological memory and motor diagrams of the human being. In adults, they awaken a corporeal intelligence that represents a valuable ally for all our physical and mental activities.

Practicing them, at any age, makes it possible to refine our motor diagrams, improve motor coordination, and rediscover the pleasure found in movement, the flexibility and finesse of a gesture, and a balanced posture. Their effects are quite stimulating and make it possible to improve the overall quality of gestural communication.

The plasticity of the nervous system, stimulated by these primitive movements, will in fact generate new connections offering new possibilities for movement. The body diagram becomes more refined in tandem, bringing about a profound and beneficial change to the gestures that accompany our daily lives and are very profound codes of expression.

Nutripuncture, by stimulating the circulation of the vital currents that activate to adjust each primitive movement, has an ideal place here. It encourages and accelerates their integration on the cerebral level, while reinforcing the construction of the identity axis.

For those wishing to learn more, the book *La marche un mouvement vital* offers a journey to the heart of "biological gymnastics." You can also consult the website: www.langage-marche.com.

THE VOICE: SPEAKING, SINGING, CREATING VIBRATIONS

Voice quality—spoken or sung—depends on the inner landscape of each individual, a shifting choreography that mirrors our physical, psychological, and emotional balance.

The voice expresses the vitality of the body; when it is in accord with its environment, an individual's vocal register expresses all of his or her sensitivity and sensuality. This is a register we define as multidimensional because it expresses the different levels of sensory acuity of the speaker: his or her taste, hearing, inspiration, vision, and tact. To optimize the currents that feed the voice and give it—both speaking and singing—all its harmonics and emotional profile, Nutripuncture has an ideal place.

It makes it possible to achieve a vocal level that only months if not years of rigorous voice training makes it possible to master. This has been noted by numerous singing teachers, artists, and speech therapists, often faced by long and difficult reeducations, which don't always have satisfactory results. In fact, when the vital currents are weakened, the vocal apparatus, and the body as a whole, need to make a colossal effort to provide a quality vocal gesture.

It is obvious that vocal exercises are essential for developing the voice. This is indispensable technical work that requires much time, patience, and perseverance. One can refine this work, even amplify its effects, by using Nutripuncture to accompany such training. Its impact on voice timbre is remarkable and the effects of this regulation can be seen immediately!

When you propel your voice with the active support of the meridians, you benefit from numerous advantages: the voice naturally finds its proper position and generates very nourishing vibrations for both the speaker and the hearer. In this way, instead of tiring, you are recharging yourself and protecting your sound legacy while stimulating your body's vocal currents. All voice professionals can draw remarkable benefits from this: conference speakers, teachers, broadcast journalists, actors, television hosts, lawyers, singers, and so on, who are often dealing with inconvenient side effects of speaking for prolonged periods or at higher volume.

For all communication through sound, Nutripuncture therefore makes it possible:

- To free yourself from physical and mental tensions that limit the full flowering of your vocal personality, and to savor the pleasure of communicating
- To protect the laryngeal system from the problems caused by vocal stress
- To promote the dynamic potential of the unexpressed qualities of the human voice, providing the body with its entire sound-making capability
- To attune your voice with your body in order to place all its resources at your body's service
- To become aware of the language of the body and the sensory information that is transported by its sonorous behavior

In short, taking care of your voice is another way to restore vitality to meridians suffering too much demand or which are exhausted, as well as to those that have not developed all their connections in the physiological network and reached full maturity, thus making it possible for you to perform at your best.

To hear voices that have been given new dynamism through Nutripuncture, you can visit the sites www.human-voice.com and www.human-voice.org.

First Experiments Using Functional Magnetic Resonance

When a person is centered and in tune with himself, he is in a state of well-being that makes it possible for the vital currents to connect all parts of the body, which encourages permanent feedback between the neural pole and the metabolic pole and ensures optimal body language and sonority.

In this situation, the individual is present to both herself and the immediate

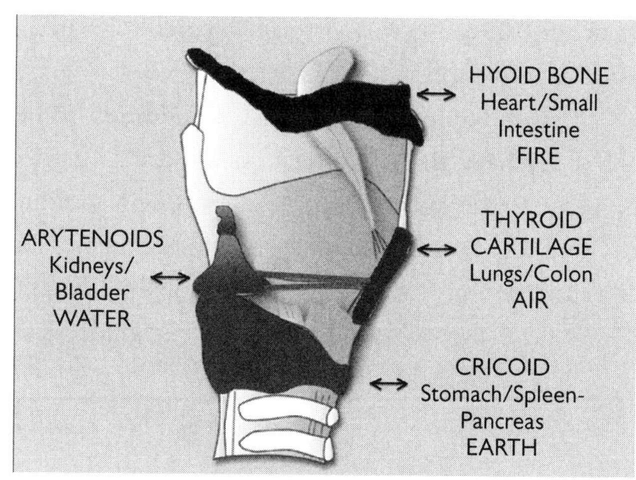

Fig. A.1. Voice quality depends on the inner landscape of each individual, a shifting choreography that mirrors our physical, psychological, and emotional balance.

surroundings, as her five senses are recording life's impressions with no interference. She can express herself without imposing herself, and at the same time can welcome others expressions without being overwhelmed by or overwhelming them. Everyone has certainly observed at one time or another that this kind of behavior tends to "contaminate" in a positive way the people with whom such a person is relating. In fact, the outlook, posture, and voice of a fulfilled individual, someone in a state of well-being, has the extraordinary power "to tune in to" the individuals with whom he or she interacts.

The consistently observed correspondence between the circulation of the vital currents, posture, viewpoint, and voice prompted our Nutripuncture research team to try to assess what induces such a harmonious "behavioral attitude." We decided to first work on the voice to measure the impact of its vibrations on the person hearing it, using Functional Magnetic Resonance Imaging (fMRI). Functional Magnetic Resonance Imaging is a non-invasive technique that makes it possible to highlight the active cerebral regions (those displaying significant oxygen consumption) during the performance of a specific task (reading, calculating, listening, moving, and so on).

In the initial phase of the study, we observed that by using a simple Associative Nutripuncture protocol, the voice improved; that is, an increase in its harmonic qualities and vibrations could be observed. Often the pitch of the voice would move a full tone or a halftone; it would also become clearer, and the speaker noted that tensions in the larynx region had vanished. This improvement was increased yet further by using a Sequential Nutripuncture protocol that made it possible to integrate cellular memories (probably tied to epigenesis) that had been interfering with behavior and sound production.*

A voice improved in this way, in addition to becoming more pleasant, both for the speaker and the listener, offers the ability to keep the listener's attention more alert. While a voice (speaking or singing) can present features that hardly go unnoticed in certain situations—such as an artist singing before an audience, giving an exceptional concert—this is unfortunately quite rare. We therefore recorded a person's improved (or, as we term it, "upgraded") voice after Nutripuncture and

*The different protocols used in this research have been described in detail in the book *La voce dei 5 sensi,* recently published in Italy.

evaluated its effect on another person listening to the recording. The first evaluations clearly indicated:

Certain vital currents of the individual who heard the upgraded voice, even when severely weakened, spontaneously recovered some vitality during the auditory stimulation.

Motor coordination and proprioception (unconscious awareness of physical movement and spatial orientation) improved.

Some osteopathic blockages vanished in real time.

We immediately thought that the upgraded voice must certainly be having an overall impact on the entire organism, the brain in particular, which could be evaluated not only indirectly (on the behavioral level or with tests), but also through methods that observe cerebral activity. We examined a test subject, who was listening to voice recordings, using fMRI, which recorded cerebral activity (one image every three seconds).

The fMRI images indicate which cerebral areas were involved during the testing, and which were not active prior to stimulation. It should be pointed out that the brain always exhibits a certain basic activity; however, the fMRI only highlights the active areas that become specifically engaged. In fact, our study intended to show how the upgraded voice activated cerebral areas that a normal voice does not stimulate.

The experiment was broken into four phases:

1. *In a recording studio:* A sample of a singer's natural speaking and singing voice was recorded after warming up. The individual was next given Nutris to obtain the upgraded voice, and a second recording was made.*
2. *In the laboratory:* The four recordings (speaking and singing voice, natural and upgraded) were cut into twelve-second intervals. The different pieces were then randomly recombined to avoid possible interference (due to a

*The time span between the first and second recordings was just several minutes long, as the trace element complexes in the Nutris provide an impulse, probably electromagnetic in nature, which has an almost immediate effect, although of brief duration. There are no grounds for believing the change was induced by other factors. In consideration of a possible placebo effect, we would like to explicitly state that an erroneous combination of the Nutris taken does not generate improvement of the voice and can even cause a temporary lowering of overall vitality.

spontaneous activation of the brain) and to be sure that the activations were actually generated by the upgraded voice.

3. *During the fMRI test:* The recordings (in which the singing and speaking, and natural and upgraded voices were linked together randomly) were played ten times to the subject, whose reactions were measured by fMRI.
4. *Construction of the images:* All the separate images obtained this way (including reactions to the singing and speaking voice, normal and upgraded) were added together to obtain a single image.

Although this was only a preliminary study, which needs further investigation (such studies are now underway), the results are quite encouraging because the images show that, compared to normal voices, the upgraded singing and speaking voices activated new cerebral areas.

If the ongoing studies conform our hypotheses with statistically significant findings, we can state we have found a new way, a new "instrument" that can be used in a number of fields, from teaching to rehabilitation.

APPENDIX B

Resources

NOW THAT YOU HAVE the basic information about Nutripuncture, further understanding can only be achieved by experiencing it. The resources presented here make it possible for you to directly order and try the Nutris for yourself. You can also gain more in-depth advice regarding actualizing your potential vitality by contacting a Nutripuncture practitioner near you. The authors further invite you to learn about Nutripuncture in a workshop.

TO ORDER NUTRIS

The trace element complexes used in Nutripuncture (Nutri Yin–Nutri Yang and the Nutris from 01–38) are nutritional supplements and can be found in health stores and online at www.getmynutri.com or by calling (877) 438-5702. Getmynutri is the importer of Nutripuncture products from France in the United States and Canada.

PRACTITIONERS

For more information or to locate a practitioner, go to **www.nutripuncture.com**.

TRAINING

By Andrew R. Heimann, AP, L.Ac.,
MSTOM, Nutripuncture Teacher

Nutripuncture is a tool that enables us to recognize our own senses and channels. When this recognition occurs, we can experience freedom. In order to understand the expansive and complex theoretical basis of Nutripuncture, it is necessary for the practitioner of Nutripuncture to experience the energetic shifts that the theory describes and explains.

This book offers invaluable theoretical knowledge of the basic principles that comprise Nutripuncture theory and practice, including the states of: 1) positive yin-yang; 2) sensory and cognitive identity; 3) anchoring in space and time; 4) spatial orientation; and 5) the expression of masculine and feminine energies. However, if the practitioner is not capable of experiencing these states energetically, this theoretical knowledge remains merely superficial, lacking the experiential understanding requisite for its proper implementation. Reading the book without also practicing and experiencing the energetic motions it traces is analogous to reading books about what a sunrise looks like, without actually having seen one firsthand. The experience of the phenomena described in this book is everything.

Accordingly, teaching Nutripuncture is one of the most challenging and rewarding experiences. It is a singularly complicated endeavor because teaching Nutripuncture aims to marry the principal, theoretical knowledge with its corresponding practical, experiential knowledge. When the marriage is successful, the insight gained into the nature of Nutripuncture and its possibilities is boundless.

This experiential knowledge begins once the teacher works with students to enable them to recognize their positive yin-yang state. This can be challenging. A person must be able to determine the identity of his or her own meridians and senses, and recognize these pathways as his or her own and not those of another. We can see from several of the sequences mentioned throughout the book that this often does not occur. Frequently, a person determines that his identity is in actuality his parent's identity or recognizes that he has information that is disturbing this particular recognition. When this information is not unique and "on" his identity, function cannot occur properly.

In my experiences as a practitioner and teacher, I am continually astonished at the ramifications of not being on one's own identity. When we are on another's identity, our core foundational beliefs of the existence of our self, along with the intake of information conveyed through the five senses, cannot be our own information or our own experience. Our core beliefs about who we are and how we relate to every other aspect of existence are fundamentally distorted. This realization can be overwhelming and frightening for some students, but for most this will be liberating. It provides the tools for becoming fearless. The clearer our recognition of our own self, the clearer our recognition of what we are not.

Following the adoption of the state of positive yin-yang, vitality requires that we be present. To establish ourselves as present, we must anchor ourselves in the "now," that is, in present time-space. We are only where we are right now. We exist now and here only, not three years ago, not where we used to live, nor where and when we wish to be. Our exchange of information, sending and receiving, only occurs in the now. Organ and meridian communication, our connection to heaven and earth, our environment, and so on, constitute living connections that demand constant open communication. The exchange of information taking place operates like a computer on a network that needs constant communication to stay synchronized with everything else on the network. If the computer is not synchronized, it cannot accept the data exchange properly, and it loses its connection to the whole. When we are not present in space and time, we lose connection to life itself. Therefore, our connection to space is important. Imagine traveling with a GPS in the United States, but with GPS maps that place us in France. We would not navigate well at all. If we are not present to ourselves, the information we process is distorted and invites disease and disorientation.

When we attain and can maintain the flow of positive yin-yang, along with beginning to recognize what it truly means to be on our identity and to function in the present, we can begin to sense our connection to everything else in a more profound and provocative way. We can then begin to explore the constant interplay of our three-dimensional relationships with the external world, as well as the constant adjustments affecting these relationships.

Finally, teaching Nutripuncture involves exploring the expressions of the male and female energies as they influence every part of human beings. Learning to sense subtle differences between the male and female energies that infuse different parts of the human anatomy opens the student to the complexities and nuances of the energetic patterns and networks that permeate our being. Then, we can begin to recognize this experience in others.

Once students have manifested these five principles, we can perhaps say they have reached the basic experiential level of humanity: to exist freely and be able to recognize others as existing freely. How can we reveal another's identity and freedom if we haven't tasted and actualized this ourselves? This is what Nutripuncture aims to accomplish.

The challenges of teaching and learning Nutripuncture point to the importance of attending and actively participating in Nutripuncture workshops. These provide the opportunity for students to gain the crucial knowledge and competency from a teacher with extensive theoretical and experiential knowledge. They facilitate the proper recognition of the five states and the corresponding energetic interplay of the individual and universe. Workshops taught by a wide variety of teachers experienced in Nutripuncture are offered throughout the United States and Europe.

In the United States: see www.nutripuncture.com, or e-mail: contact@nutripuncture.com. Andrew Heimann can be contacted at: asknutripuncture@gmail.com.

In France, the Association Médicale Internationale Nutripuncture Europe (A.M.I.N.E.) offers Nutripuncture training for health professionals. The association also offers internships, open to the public, to enable providers to better grasp the role played by the meridians in individual psychophysical dynamics.

APPENDIX C

Testimonials

THE TESTIMONIALS presented here are not intended to be demonstrative but simply to express the experience some individuals have had with Nutripuncture. In the scientific realm, medical therapies are based on "proof of effectiveness," meaning data that is statistically significant. Nutripuncture does not view itself as a substitute for standard medical therapy, which represents what has been demonstrated scientifically with its own insights and dark areas.

Nutripuncture is an approach that focuses on the complex dynamics of life. It should not be viewed as a therapy for fighting disease as much as a means for empowering individuals to draw from their own inner resources and to activate the body's information, which has often been short-circuited by stress, yet is essential for the body's ability to regulate itself. We are aware that we are on the threshold of a life science that will certainly open new horizons in the research on human potential.

Nutripuncture's Contribution to Dealing with Grief

I lost my grandfather in March 2002. This came as a huge shock to me and I was unable to mourn him properly. For five years I was like a soul in torment, ceaselessly thinking of him, crying constantly, and still living as if he was always still at my side. This situation became untenable and I was truly unhappy. As a final resort, as all the prior methods I tried failed, I turned to Dr. T. He recommended I take a Nutripuncture sequence twice a day for a month. I followed a specific protocol for "digesting" my *grandfather's death and recognizing my origin and psychophysical identity.* The results were spectacular. I can live today with my mind at ease. This testimony is my way of thanking Dr. T. and, most importantly, the very effective help I got from the Nutris, help that changed my life.*

Karine F., Geneva, Switzerland

Nutripuncture's Contribution to Combating Depression

Over a period of several years my depression had become chronic. Anti-anxiety drugs, anti-depressants, psychologists—nothing stopped my relapses, which became deeper and deeper.

I often visualized the interior of my body as a chimney filled with soot. Everything was dark and black. I could scrub as hard as I could in the shower, but I always felt dirty.

When I had a relapse, the past suddenly burst back like a flash in my mind. I had been a victim of incest! When I was still a little girl my big brother would molest me and threaten me with his fist not to say anything to papa and mama . . . this was a real shock and caused a lot of pain.

But here again, although the cause for my depression was fully known, traditional medicine and psychotherapy had no result.

To help me out of this daily hell, a friend told me about Dr. V. I was somewhat skeptical but I really wanted to get free of this. I followed his advice very conscientiously and I ingested the Nutris he recommended.†

I felt better very quickly; I might even say—though this is surprising—immediately. Then in the span of three months my depression vanished. The feeling of being dirty that had flooded me also vanished. Now I feel "clean," with all stains washed away. I have buried the past and finally have plans for the future. Finally I exist!

Françoise B., Lyon, France

---

*The Nutripuncture protocol mentioned here consists of three sequences: acknowledging our genetic origin (see page 146); adopting our body (see page 146); becoming aware of death and acknowledging the cellular cycle (see page 148).

†The Sequential Nutripuncture for rape was used here (see page 166).

Nutripuncture's Assistance against Depression Following a Rape

A girlfriend recommended I go see Dr. G. because I had been having anxiety attacks since childhood. I never really knew what the profound cause was and I saw psychologists and psychiatrists. The pharmaceutical treatments I was prescribed helped lessen my anxieties a little but I often had relapses. The fact that I was raped by an uncle might have been a triggering factor, but discussing it with my psychotherapists never really brought me any relief.

In fact, while I knew it happened I could not accept it and believe it. It felt like a nightmare that had happened next to me and inside me at the same time: a sensation that is very hard to put into words.

So I decided to go see this doctor, while telling myself, "I will see what happens in any case." And I did see!!! I told him about my history with this uncle and he suggested a specific protocol, which, he explained to me, would reactivate the vital currents to recover my integrity and the feeling of being comfortable in my own skin, and to acknowledge facts that I did not want to integrate consciously, although I knew what they were.

I really have to tell you that the two sequences I took for a month had remarkable effects. Today I feel liberated from this burden; I am no longer taking any medications, not even any Nutris. I even recommended this same protocol to a friend who found equally satisfying results.*

It is a pleasure to tell this story and I hope it can help other women who have lost their integrity, because what they have experienced can be a real tragedy.

ISABELLE I., BRUSSELS, BELGIUM

Nutripuncture's Contribution to Dealing with a Physical Trauma

I was shopping when a dog attached to a pole waiting for its owner suddenly lunged at me, pulling on his leash. I fell down without really noticing it. There was blood

*These two Nutripuncture sequences were for rape (see page 166) and forgiveness (see page 167).

on my face and most importantly a pain by my left knee that prevented me from getting back up and then from walking. The doctor I consulted only gave me anti-inflammatories, and after a month my condition had still not improved. I still had trouble walking, getting out of a car, or getting up from a chair. This alarmed me quite a bit because I was scared nothing could be done: in one fell swoop, at sixty years of age, I felt old and handicapped. A casual friend told me a similar story and about the Nutris he had given his wife after a bone trauma. Because they were only food supplements, I gladly tried them. After two days, the pain was reduced by half, I could walk more easily, and I had recovered my usual good spirits. After fifteen days I was walking normally. Bravo the Nutris.*

CLAUDIA M., SAN FRANCISCO, CALIFORNIA

Nutripuncture's Assistance in Treating Problems with Swallowing

I have always had problems swallowing since childhood. One day, while driving my car, the candy I was eating got stuck in my throat. I was gripped by a terrible panic and I felt like I was suffocating. I stopped to find help immediately. Fortunately there was a café close by, and once I had parked, I grabbed a bottle of water standing on the counter. The barman, who knew me, understood my problem at once and slapped me on the back. What relief: my throat was open again and I could breathe! I next went to the hospital where they took some x-rays. The piece of candy had actually gone down the wrong tube and fallen into my lung. They decided to give me antibiotics until it no longer showed up on x-rays.

This accident not only revealed how serious my problem with swallowing was, but it also triggered a strong sense of anxiety because the risk of another "accident" was always present. In fact, even though it had always bothered me, I had never looked for ways to improve my swallowing. But following this incident, I was truly motivated to resolve my "handicap."

When I told this to a friend who was a doctor, he urgently advised me to reeducate my throat using specific exercises and to take Nutripuncture sequences, which he

*This is the Sequential Nutripuncture protocol for bone trauma (see page 167).

used for his patients. I began by using the Nutris because I had not found enough time to also do the exercises.*

After a month and a half taking these sequences, I passed my deglutition test perfectly. My throat was more relaxed, my neck muscles had better tone, and my locution was improved. Today, I feel freed and these problems that had owned me since childhood are nothing but a bad memory.

Piera D., Turin, Italy

Nutripuncture's Value for Resolving Family Conflicts

I have always had difficult relations with my daughter. All my attempts and steps to find reconciliation failed. I kept running into non-comprehension. I could not come up with the solution I wanted and this caused me enormous suffering.

I opened up about this to my practitioner, a Nutripuncture specialist. While hearing me out, he highlighted the vital currents that were involved in my distress and recommended some personalized Nutripuncture combinations, which I began taking the next day.† After several weeks my daughter saw how I had changed and became intrigued. Since taking the Nutris, I have been more stable and at ease, and this has helped me find just the right words for talking with her. I think that my new attitude will bring her to a better sense of well-being.

I owe finding my way out of this imbroglio in which we were caught to the Nutri supplements; I can now regard the future with calm and tranquillity.

Josette R., Paris, France

Nutripuncture's Contribution to Family Dynamics (Mother-Daughter Identifications)

I consulted Dr. G. after my daughter left home because I felt abandoned and had the impression that I had been straight out "robbed." I remember that when I saw

---

*This is a specific Nutripuncture sequence (Adult Deglutition) used by certain practitioners (dentists, osteopaths, speech therapists) to reeducate so-called infantile deglutition:

For Men: 33, 16, 36, 27, 10 + 33, 21, 26, 16, 10

For Women: 33, 16, 35, 27, 10 + 33, 28, 26, 16, 10

†This was a specific Associative Nutripuncture combination made "to order" to drain the terrain of the person in question.

Dr. G. I told him word for word: "My daughter deceived me, she left with a man, I want to kill him!" I described what was a dramatic situation for me. Dr G., who had much more detachment, simply told me: "Madame, it is not that serious. It is simply the complete fusion with your daughter that is making you experience a kind of reversed Oedipus complex. Your discomfort is the opportunity to recognize it and restore the vital currents that have gone off course—which is what is responsible for your distress—to their proper place. He suggested I try a specific sequence and this calmed me down and made me feel as if a huge burden had been lifted from my shoulders. I had the impression that when I thought about my daughter it was as if she was detached from my body and all at once we were two separate individuals.*

I followed his very helpful advice and ingested the Nutris for thirty days and went back to see him a month later. I no longer had any desire to kill that man, nor anybody else. I had finally found my position as a mother and freed my daughter with whom I have been able to establish less possessive and calmer communication. Today I tell myself my attitude was truly incredible: how can anyone delude themselves to this extent and construct unhealthy relationships which sometimes keep them prisoner all their life?

Sandra M., Milan, Italy

Nutripuncture's Contribution for Treating Infertility

I had been trying to have a baby for several years and, despite three in-vitro fertilizations, no baby had yet arrived. My tests were apparently normal and the doctors did not know why it was not working. It was a long-time friend, to whom I had confided my problems, who recommended I call an acupuncturist who practiced Nutripuncture. This person advised me to have an extensive chart drawn up with another practitioner closer to home. However, while I was waiting to make an appointment, he suggested an overall Associative Nutripuncture protocol to save time.† So I began following his

---

*This is the specific Nutripuncture sequence for identification with the parent of the same sex (see page 156).

†This was a general Associative Nutripuncture protocol for infertility:
Nutri Yin–Nutri Yang + Nutri 28 + Nutri 24 + Nutri 33

recommendations before going to see the other acupuncturist (who I never ended up consulting) because I had no desire to be on a six-month waiting list.

I took the Nutris indicated in the protocol he gave me, and after only two months I got pregnant. This was really incredible, as I had already gone through complicated treatments as well as the in-vitro fertilizations with no results. The acupuncturist I had spoken to on the phone had simply suggested I activate the vital currents involved in feminine expression (the vital currents of the Uterus and the Breasts). I actually quickly felt a sense of relaxation I had not felt for a very long time. Is it because I recovered a certain equilibrium, felt more fulfilled, more womanly that I became pregnant? I do not know; all I know is that—it worked!

ANNICK M., STRASBOURG, FRANCE

Notes

Preface: Introducing the Authors

1. P. Nogier, *Treatise on Auriculotherapy* (Maisonneuve: Moulins-les-Metz, 1963); *The Man in the Ear* (Maisonneuve: Moulins-les-Metz, 1979); *A Practical Introduction to Auriculotherapy* (Maisonneuve: Moulins-les-Metz, 1977); *From Auriculotherapy to Auriculomedicine* (Maisonneuve: Moulins-les-Metz, 1981).

Introduction: What Is Nutripuncture?

1. F. A. Popp, *Biologie de la Lumière* (Liège, Belgium: Pietteur, 1989); V. L. Voeikov, ed., *Biophotonics and Coherent Systems in Biology* (Moscow: Moscow University Press, 2000); A. Gurwitsch, *Phenomenology and Theory of Science* (Evanston, Ill.: Northwestern University Press, 1974).

Chapter 1. Acupuncture without Needles

1. Edgar Morin, *Le paradigme perdu: la nature humaine* (Paris: Seuil, 1973).

Chapter 3. Four Vital Parameters for the Body, Four Essential Conditions for Ensuring Its Vitality

1. Alain Ehrenberg, *The Weariness of the Self* (Montreal: McGill-Queen's University Press, 2010).

Chapter 10. Getting Your Bearings and Discovering Your Body's Potential

1. Edgar Morin, *L'Homme et la mort* (Paris: Seuil, 1951).

Appendix A: Nutripuncture, an Ideal Instrument for Supporting Human Communication

1. Patrick Veret, Cristina Cuomo, *La Voix pluridimensionelle* (Micropolis, France: Des Iris, 2006).

Bibliography

Académie de médecine traditionnelle chinoise. *Précis d'acupuncture chinoise.* Peking: Éditions en langues étrangères, 1977.

Ackerman, N. W. *The Psychodynamics of Family Life.* New York: Basic Books, 1958.

Adler, A. *The Practice and Theory of Individual Psychology* (1920). London: Routledge, 1999.

Ambrosini, C., C. De Panfilis, and A. M. Willie. *La psicomotricità: corporeità e azione nella costruzione dell'identità.* Milan: Xenia, 1999.

Ameisen, J-C. *La sculpture du vivant.* Paris: Seuil, 2003.

Atlan, H., J. De Rosnay, A. Jacquard, J-M. Pelt, I. Prigogine, and T. Xuan Thuan. *Le monde s'est-il créé tout seul?* Paris: Albin Michel, 2008.

Bateson, G. *Mind and Nature.* New York: Dutton, 1979.

———. *Steps to an Ecology of Mind.* New York: Ballantine, 1985.

Berg, J. M., and S. J. Lippard. *Principles of Bioinorganic Chemistry.* Mill Valley, Calif.: University Science Books, 1994.

Bergeret, J., M. Soulé, and B. Golse. *Anthropologie du foetus.* Paris: Dunod, 2006.

Berti, A-M., and A-S. Bombi. *Psicologia dello sviluppo.* Bologna: Il Mulino, 2001.

Bion, W. R. *Apprendere dall'esperienza.* Rome: Armando Editore, 1972.

Bocchi, G., and M. Cerruti. *Origini di teorie.* Milan: Feltrinelli, 1993.

Boissin, J., and B. Canguilhem. *Les Rythmes du Vivant.* Paris: CNRS Edition, 1998.

Bottaccioli, F. *Psiconeuro endocrino immunologia.* Como, Italy: RED, 1995.

———. *Il Sistema Immunitario: la bilancia della vita.* Milan: Tecniche Nuove, 2002.

Bowlby, J. *Attaccamento e perdita.* Turin, Italy: Bollati Boringhieri, 1972.

———. *La base sicura.* Milan: Raffaello Cortina, 1988.

Brun, J. *Héraclite, le philosophe de l'éternel retour.* Paris: Seghers, 1965.

Bruner, J. S. *Le développement de l'enfant: savoir faire, savoir dire.* Paris: PUF, 1991.

———. *La mente a più dimension.* Rome: Laterza, 1988.

Burigana, F., C. Cuomo, and P. Veret. *La voce dei 5 sensi.* Milan: Carisch, 2011.

Burigana, F., and R. P. Stefani. *Chinesiologia, l'armonia segreta del corpo.* Milan: Xenia, 1998.

Caprara, G. V., and D. Cervone. *Personalità: determinanti, dinamiche, potenzialità.* Milan: Cortina, 2003.

Caprara, G. V., and A. Gennaro. *Psicologia della personalità.* Bologna: Il Mulino, 1999.

Cuomo, C. *La marche, un mouvement vital.* Paris: Dauphin, 2008.

Cyrulnick, B. *Un merveilleux malheur.* Paris: Odile Jacob, 2002.

———. *La naissance du sens.* Paris: Hachette, 1995.

———. De la parole comme une molécule. Paris: Points, 1995.

———. *Les vilains petits canards.* Paris: Odile Jacob, 2001.

Cyrulnick, B., and E. Morin. *Dialogue sur la nature humaine.* La Tour d'Aigues, France: L'Aube, 2000.

Damasio, A. R. *Emozione e coscienza.* Milan: Adelphi, 2000.

Dawson, C. *Medicina Epigenetica.* Rome: Mediterranee, 2008.

Dolto, F. *Les étapes majeures de l'enfance.* Paris: Gallimard, 1994.

Ehrenberg, A. *The Weariness of the Self: Diagnosing the History of Depression in the Contemporary Age.* Montreal: McGill-Queen's University Press, 2010.

Erickson, E. H. *Childhood and Society.* New York: Norton, 1950.

Fay, T. "The Origin of Human Movement." *American Journal of Psychiatry* 111 (March 1955): 644–52.

Foster, R., and L. Kreitzman. *I ritmi della vita.* Milan: Longanesi, 2004.

Frankl, V. E. *Un significato per l'esistenza: psicoterapia e umanismo.* Bologna: Città Nuova, 1990.

Freud, S. *La disparition du complexe d'Œdipe.* Paris: Presses Universitaires de France, 1992. First published 1924.

———. *L'organisation génitale infantile.* Paris: Presses Universitaires de France, 1991. First published 1923.

———. *Three Essays on the Theory of Sexuality.* New York: Avon, 1962.

Frölich, H. *Biological Coherence and Response to External Stimuli.* New York: Pringer-Verlag, 1988.

———. *Coherent Excitations in Biological Systems.* New York: Springer, 1983.

Fullerton, C. S., and R. J. Ursano. *Disturbo Post-traumatico da Stress.* Turin, Italy: Centro Scientifico Editore, 2001.

Gazzaniga, M. S. *Human.* Milan: Raffaello Cortina, 2009.

Gibran, K. *The Prophet.* New York: Knopf, 1965.

Goleman, D. *Emotional Intelligence.* New York: Bantam, 1995.

Goodman, R., Y. Chizmaden, and A. Shirley-Henderson. "Electromagnetic Fields and Cells," *Journal of Cellular Biochemistry* 51 (1993).

Grand, I. *The Body in Psychotherapy*. Berkeley: North Atlantic Books, 1998.

Guillé, E. *L'alchimie de la vie*. Monaco: Du Rocher, 1984.

Gurwitsch, A. *Phenomenology and Theory of Science*. Evanston, Ill.: Northwestern University Press, 1974.

———. *Problems of Mitogenetic Radiation as an Aspect of Molecular Biology*. Leningrad: Meditaina, 1968.

Heidegger, M. *Being and Time*. Albany: State University of New York Press, 1996. First published 1927.

Héraclite. *La main et l'esprit*. Paris: PUF, 1963.

Heraclitus. *Fragments*. London, New York: Penguin, 2003.

Holmes, J. *La teoria dell'attaccamento*. Milan: Raffaello Cortina, 1994.

Iacoboni, M. *I neuroni specchio*. Milan: Bollati Boringhieri, 2008.

Jablonka, E., and M. J. Lamb. *L'evoluzione in quattro dimensioni. Variazione genetica, epigenetica, comportamentale e simbolica nella storia della vita*. Turin, Italy: UTET, 2007.

James, W. *Principles of Psychology*. New York: Cosimo, 2007. First published in 1890.

Jung, C. *Psychological Types*. New York: Harcourt Brace, 1923.

———. *Les racines de la conscience*. Paris: Buchet-Chastel, 1975.

Klein, M. *Sulla teoria dell'angoscia e del senso di colpa* (*Scritti* 1921–1958). Milan: Bollati Boringhieri, 1978.

Labreque, G., and M. Sirois. *Chronopharmacologie, rythmes biologiques et administration des medicaments*. Montreal: Les Presses de l'Université de Montréal, 2004.

Lakovsky, G. *L'oscillation cellulaire*. Paris: Doin, 1931.

———. *La science du Bonheur*. Paris: Gauthier Villars, 1930.

———. *Le secret de la vie*. Paris: Gauthier Villars, 1925.

Lavier, J. A. *Bio-énérgétique chinoise*. Paris: Maloine, 1983.

Lebarbier, A. *Acupunctute pratique*. Paris: Maisonneuve, 1975.

Lewin, K. *Principi di psicologia topologica*. Florence: Os, 1970.

———. *Teoria dinamica della personalità*. Florence: Giunti Barbera, 1965.

Lipton, B. H. *Biology of Belief*. New York: Hay House, 2008.

Liu, F., and G. Y. Huang. "Advances of Studies on the Biophysical and Biochemical Properties of Meridians." *Zen Ci Yan Jiu* 32, no. 4 (August 2007): 281–84.

Lowen, A. *La depressione e il corpo*. Rome: Astrolabio, 1980. First published 1972.

———. *Il linguaggio del corpo*. Milan: Feltrinelli, 2004.

Magnin, P. *Des rythmes de vie aux rythmes scolaires*. Paris: PUF, 1993.

Manghi, S. *Attraverso Bateson*. Milan: Raffaello Cortina, 1988.

Maturana, H. R. *Tree of Knowledge*. Boston: Shambhala, 1992.

Maturana, H. R., and F. J. Varela. *Autopoiesi e cognizione*. Padua, Italy: Marsilio, 1985.

McClintock, B. "Chromosome Organization and Genic Expression." *Cold Spring Harbor Symposia on Quantitative Biology* 16 (1951): 13–47.

Merleau-Ponty, M. *La struttura del comportamento.* Milan: Bompiani, 1963. First published 1942.

Montuori, A., and I. Conti. *Dal dominio alla partecipazione.* Milan: Etas, 1997.

Morin, E. *La Complexité humaine.* Paris: Flammarion, 1994.

———. *Cultura e barbarie europee.* Milan: Raffaello Cortina, 2006.

———. *L'Homme et la mort.* Paris: Seuil, 1951.

———. *La Méthode 5: L'humanité de l'humanité, l'identité humaine.* Paris: Seuil, Nouvelle édition, 2001.

———. *La Méthode 6: Éthique.* Paris: Seuil, Nouvelle edition, 2004.

———. *Il paradigma perduto: la natura umana.* Milan: Bompiani, 1973.

———. *Le paradigme perdu: la nature humaine.* Paris: Seuil, 1973.

———. *Relier les connaissances.* Paris: Seuil, 1999.

———. *Science avec Conscience.* Paris: Fayard, 1982.

———. *Les sept savoirs nécessaires à l'éducation du future.* Paris: Seuil, 2000.

———. *La testa ben fatta. Riforma dell'insegnamento e riforma del pensiero.* Milan: Raffaello Cortina, 2000.

Morin, E., and A. Martini. *Educare gli educatori. Una riforma del pensiero per la democrazia cognitive.* Bologna: EdUP, 1999.

Niccolò, A-M. *Adolescenza e violenza.* Rome: Il Pensiero Scientifico Editore, 2009.

Nogier, P. *From Auriculotherapy to Auriculomedicine.* Maisonneuve: Moulins-les-Metz, 1981.

———. *The Man in the Ear.* Maisonneuve: Moulins-les-Metz, 1979.

———. *A Practical Introduction to* Auriculotherapy. Maisonneuve: Moulins-les-Metz, 1977.

———. *Treatise on Auriculotherapy.* Maisonneuve: Moulins-les-Metz, 1963.

Olimpiade, L. *Nuove possibilità per il trattamento delle obesità mediante la somministrazione calibrata di oligoelementi.* Rome: Università Roma Tor Vergata, 2006–2007.

Oliverio, A. *Geografia della mente.* Milan: Raffaello Cortina, 2008.

Paris, J. *Contesto sociale e disturbi di personalità.* Milan: Raffaello Cortina, 1997.

Parquer, Y., and P. Veret. *Traité de Nutripuncture.* Micropolis, France: DesIris, 2005.

Pigozzi, L. *A nuda voce.* Turin, Italy: Antigone Edizioni, 2008.

Popp, F. A. *Biologie de la lumière.* Liege, Belgium: Pietteur, 1989.

———. *La teoria dei biofotoni.* Montreal: IPSA, 1985.

Prigogine, I. "L'esplorazione della complessità." In *La sfida della complessità.* Edited by Gianluca Bocchi and Mauro Ceruti. Milan: Feltrinelli, 1997.

———. *Le leggi del caos.* Rome: Laterza, 1993.

Purves, D. *Neuroscienze.* Turin, Italy: Zanichelli, 2005.

Reveillard, J. P. *Immunologie.* Brussels. De Boeck, 1998.

Rizzolati, G. and C. Sinigaglia. *So quel che fai.* Milan: Raffaello Cortina, 2006.

Rocca, B. *Medicina Quantistica Molecolare.* Milan: Tecniche Nuove, 2008.

Schindler, O., G. Righini, and C. Giordano. *Biologia della musica.* Turin, Italy: Omega, 1999.

Spaggiari, P., and C. Tribbia. *Medicina quantistica.* Milan: Tecniche Nuove, 2002.

Spitz, R. A. *De la naissance à la parole.* Paris: PUF, 1968.

Stern, D. N. *Journal d'un bébé.* Paris: Calmann-Lévy, 1992.

———. *La nascita del Sé.* Rome: Laterza, 1989.

Tassinari, G. *Le basi fisologiche della percezione e del movimento.* Bologna: Il Mulino, 1999.

Terzani, T. *Lettere contro la Guerra.* Milan: TEA, 2008.

Thirion, M. *Les compétences du nouveau-né.* Paris: Albin Michel, 2002.

Trojani, F. *L'homme électromagnétique.* Paris: Dervy, 2008.

Varela, F. J. *Ponti sottili.* Milan: Neri Pozzi Editori, 1998.

Varela, F. J., E. Thompson, and E. Rosch. *The Embodied Mind, Cognitive Science and Human Experience.* Boston: MIT Press, 1992.

Veret, P. *La médecine énergétique.* Monaco: Du Rocher, 1981.

Veret, P., and C. Cuomo. *La Voix pluridimensionelle.* Micropolis, France: Des Iris, 2006.

Vidal, C. *Le cerveau évolue-t-il au cours de la vie?* Paris: Le Pommier, 2009.

———. *Hommes, femmes, avons nous le même cerveau?* Paris: Le Pommier, 2007.

Voeikov, V. L., F. A. Popp, and L. V. Beloussov. *Biophotonics and Coherent Systems in Biology.* Moscow: Moscow University Press, 2000.

Voisin, H. *L'acupuncture du praticien.* Paris: Maloine, 1979.

Vygotskij, L. *Pensiero e linguaggio.* Florence: Giunti Barbera, 1966. First published 1934.

Winnicott, D. W. *The Child, the Family, and the Outside World.* New York: Perseus, 1992.

———. *La mère suffisamment bonne.* Paris: Payot, 1996.

———. *Playing and Reality.* London: Routledge, 2005. First published 1975.

———. *Sviluppo affettivo e ambiente.* Rome: Armando Editore, 1970.

Zavattini, G. C. *La trasmissine transgenerazionale delle emozioni e la funzione del Sé autoriflessiv, Atti dell'Accademia di Scienze morali e politiche.* Napoli: Giannini, 1997.

Index

Page numbers in *italics* refer to illustrations.